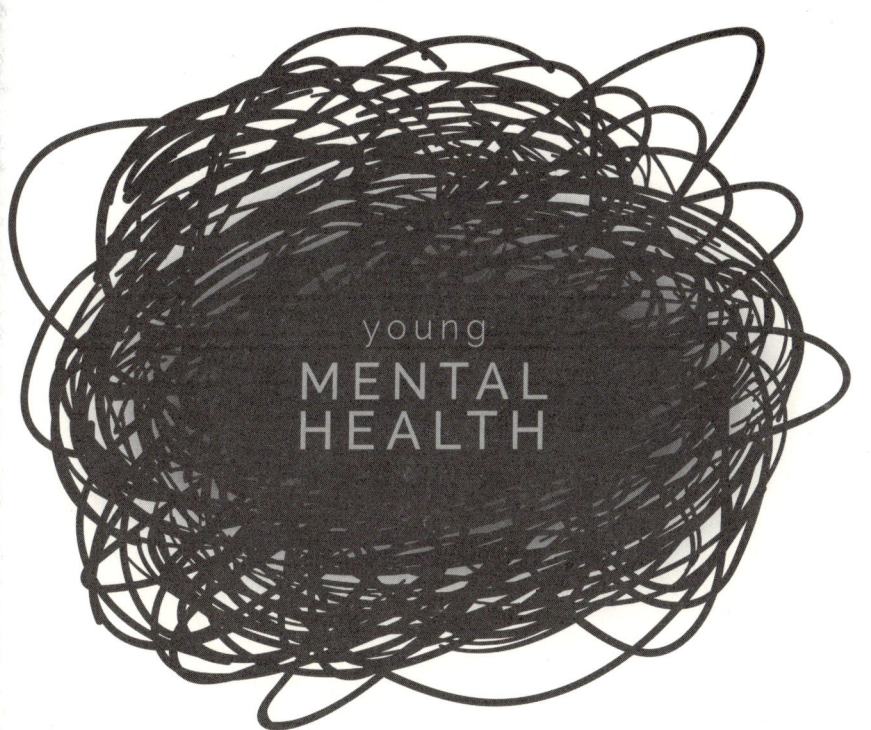

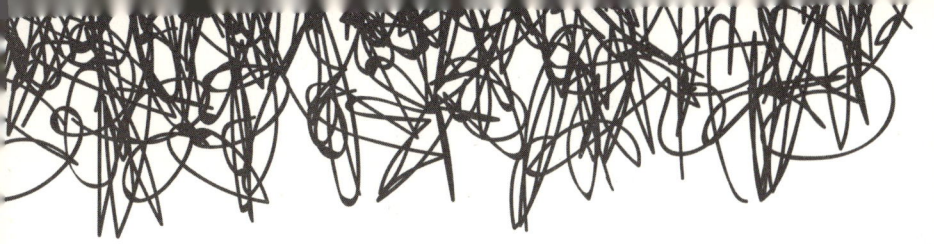

young
MENTAL HEALTH

AMRITA TRIPATHI
MEERA HARAN ALVA

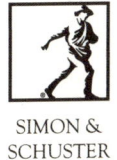

SIMON &
SCHUSTER

London • New York • Sydney • Toronto • New Delhi

A CBS COMPANY

First published in India by Simon & Schuster India, 2020
A Viacom CBS company

Copyright © Amrita Tripathi, 2020
Art: Ishita Mehra, Solo, Oz, Kishore Mohan and Adwaita Das

The right of Amrita Tripathi to be identified as author of
this work has been asserted by her in accordance with
Section 57 of the Copyright Act 1957.

1 3 5 7 9 10 8 6 4 2

Simon & Schuster India
818, Indraprakash Building,
21, Barakhamba Road,
New Delhi 110001

www.simonandschuster.co.in

Paperback ISBN: 978-93-86797-46-9
eBook ISBN: 978-93-86797-47-6

Typeset in India by Mridu Agarwal, Simon & Schuster, New Delhi

Printed and bound in India by Replika Press Pvt. Ltd.

Simon & Schuster India is committed to sourcing paper that is made from wood grown in sustainable forests and support the Forest Stewardship Council,® the leading international forest certification organisation. Our books displaying the FS ®C logo are
printed on FSC® certified paper.

No part of this publication may be reproduced, transmitted or stored in a retrieval system, in any form or by any means, electronic, mechanical, photocopying, recording or otherwise, without the prior permission of the publisher.

This book is sold subject to the condition that it shall not, by way of trade or otherwise, be lent, resold, hired out, or otherwise circulated, without the publisher's prior consent, in any form of binding or cover other than that in which it is published.

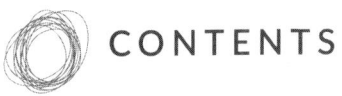

CONTENTS

Foreword	**1**
Child and Adolescent Psychiatrist Dr Amit Sen	1
Introduction and About the Book	**4**
Amrita Tripathi	5
Moving in the Right Direction	**12**
Meera Haran Alva	12
PART 1	**20**
Chapter 1	22
The Context: Why does Young Mental Health Matter?	**23**
Chapter 2	28
What's Stressing Out India's Kids?	**29**
- Interview with Dr Amit Sen	30
- Art by Kishore Mohan	37
Chapter 3	52
In Their Own Words	**53**
Learning to Heal: Story and Art by Ishita Mehra	54
Chapter 4	56
On ADHD	**57**
- Words by Dr Amit Sen	57
- Art by Kishore Mohan	61
- In Their Own Words by Dr Sen	62
Chapter 5	68
Sharing the Struggle	**69**
- Interview with Paras Sharma	70

Chapter 6

On Bullying

- Art by Solo
- Words by Dr Amit Sen
- Affirmation by Adwaita Das

Chapter 7

In Their Own Words

- Battling Fear, Depression and the Pressure to Always be Good by Anwesh Pokkuluri
- Affirmation by Adwaita Das

Chapter 8

Suicide Prevention

- In Their Own Words by Manisha Chachra
- Creating the Space to Seek Help by Kamna Chhibber

Chapter 9

In Their Own Words

- What Helps: Words and Art by Ishita Mehra

Chapter 10

In Their Own Words: Youth Speak

- Surveys on Youth and Mental Health
- Words and Art by Young Mental Health Advocate Ananya Dhanuka

Chapter 11

In Their Own Words

- Could this be Home? Story and Art by Solo
- Affirmation by Adwaita Das

PART 2

Chapter 12

Understanding Young India

- Interview with Pattie Gonsalves
- Interview with Tanuja Babre

Chapter 13	154
In Their Own Words	**155**
-Aftermath: Words and Art by Oz	156
Chapter 14	158
FAQ's and A Practical Handbook for Parents	**159**
- What is Normal? Parenting FAQ's and Understanding Therapy by Meera Haran Alva	159
Chapter 15	192
Young Depression and Anxiety	**193**
- Toolboxes for Parents and Case Illustrations by Meera Haran Alva	204
- Child Sexual Abuse Signs to Watch Out For	223
- Affirmation by Adwaita Das	224
Chapter 16	230
In Their Own Words	**231**
- What I Learned from Trying to Cope with My Borderline Personality Diagnosis: Story and Art by Solo	231
Chapter 17	232
Eating Disorders and Body Image Disorder	**233**
- In Their Own Words: Overcoming an Eating Disorder (Anonymous)	
- Myths and Facts by Smriti Joshi and Pragya Lodha	233
Chapter 18	254
Mental Health and Students	**254**
- Promoting Mental Health in the Student Population by Dr Samir Parikh and Kamna Chhibber	255
- Five Tips to Deal with Exam-Related Stress by Dr Samir Parikh and Kamna Chhibberr	264
- In Their Own Words: Young Mental Health Advocate Yash Shah	266

Helplines in India

Acknowledgements

Endnotes

FOREWORD BY DR AMIT SEN

I remember when I decided to pursue psychiatry after becoming a doctor and announced it to my family — my *Didima/Nani* (maternal grandmother), who was amongst one of my favourite persons, was aghast. 'After all these years of hard work and toil, you want to become a *pagoler dactar* (Bangla for "lunatic's doctor")?!' Back in the 1980s, psychiatry was a poor choice to make from every angle, whether it was social status, financial returns, or the cynicism with which it was viewed amongst our own medical fraternity.

A lot has changed since then, not least in the way mental health problems have sky-rocketed, but much more in the way the world has started looking at it. The notion that mental illness can only happen to another person or family and not me or mine, is beginning to shift significantly. Rather than seeing it as an incomprehensible experience happening to the other, people have started seeing it as a realistic possibility in their own lives. Media articles and stories, testimonials from famous people, cinema, literature, poetry and music have all started expressing and highlighting it as a real life experience that could happen to anybody. Mental health professionals too have started shifting their stance increasingly, from perceiving and interpreting mental illness from a purely medical and expert-driven model to a psychosocial model that is collaborative and respectful. There is a growing understanding that trying to manage mental health difficulties in hospitals and clinics by experts is going to only touch the tip of the iceberg, and that we need to reach out to the larger community to make a broader and deeper impact.

While there have been encouraging strides in adult mental health, including the new Mental Health Care Act, 2017 in India, which is sensitive, inclusive and

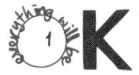

empowering of people suffering from mental illnesses, the children of the country have not got their due. The laws of the land, including the Juvenile Justice Act (JJ Act) 2015, and Protection of Children from Sexual Offences (POCSO) 2012, which are guided by principles of child rights and protection, are comprehensive and robust, but their implementation is woefully lacking or short-sighted and punitive. The reason for this is a poor understanding of children's needs and the abject lack of resources, I believe. The fact that healthy mental (and physical) development of a child is a dynamic process that depends upon the complex interplay between their temperament, their ever-changing needs as they grow and the turbulent world around them, is a challenging concept to grasp. The strife-ridden socio-political imbroglio that threatens to enter our homes today, coupled with the changing family structure, urbanisation, intense competitiveness in education, the impact of social media and the prevailing uncertainty that all this creates only makes it that much more difficult to understand.

Is it any wonder that one in four young people are now known to suffer from clinical depression before they turn 18, that cutting oneself has become a common method of expressing distress, that substance use is rampant in schools and colleges as a way of coping with stress, that body image and eating habits occupy young peoples' minds in obsessive forms, that confusion surrounding gender and sexuality makes the young and the old take up polarised and litigious positions?

In India, the situation is particularly fractious, as we are confronted with disturbing events and statistics that shake the foundation of our collective belief that we are a family-oriented and child-centric society. How can we explain that, as a country, we have one of the highest rates of child sexual abuse

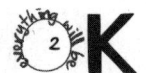

if we are indeed protective of our children?! India also has one of the highest suicide rates amongst young people in the world; suicide is the number one cause of death in young people between the ages of 15 and 29 (38 per 1,00,000).[1]

To say that the scenario is alarming would be an understatement. If we really hope that this young generation will take us to a promising future, all stakeholders will need to do something transformative to help them achieve it. What we need is a movement that will challenge institutions, revolutionise systems and change the very language that we use to speak to and about our children.

In this context, this book is timely and much needed. The fact that it has attempted to look at child and adolescent mental health from different lenses, both expert and non-expert, is refreshing, and provides the reader various choices to align to or learn from. While it has taken from research at esteemed institutions, it has also sensitively explored the story of an adolescent struggling with sexuality and depression. Innovative models created by young therapists and community based interventions reaching out to thousands and more are insightful and exciting. The authors have been able to successfully weave together a tapestry of ideas, experiences and evolving models of prevention and care that are relevant and inspiring. Their desire to inform and passion to transform is palpable.

The biggest achievement of this book, I believe, is that it can arouse the curiosity in a sceptical adolescent as much as it can engage the cynical professional. I sincerely hope that it reaches tens of thousands, young and old, who need to go through this compelling book.

March 2020
New Delhi

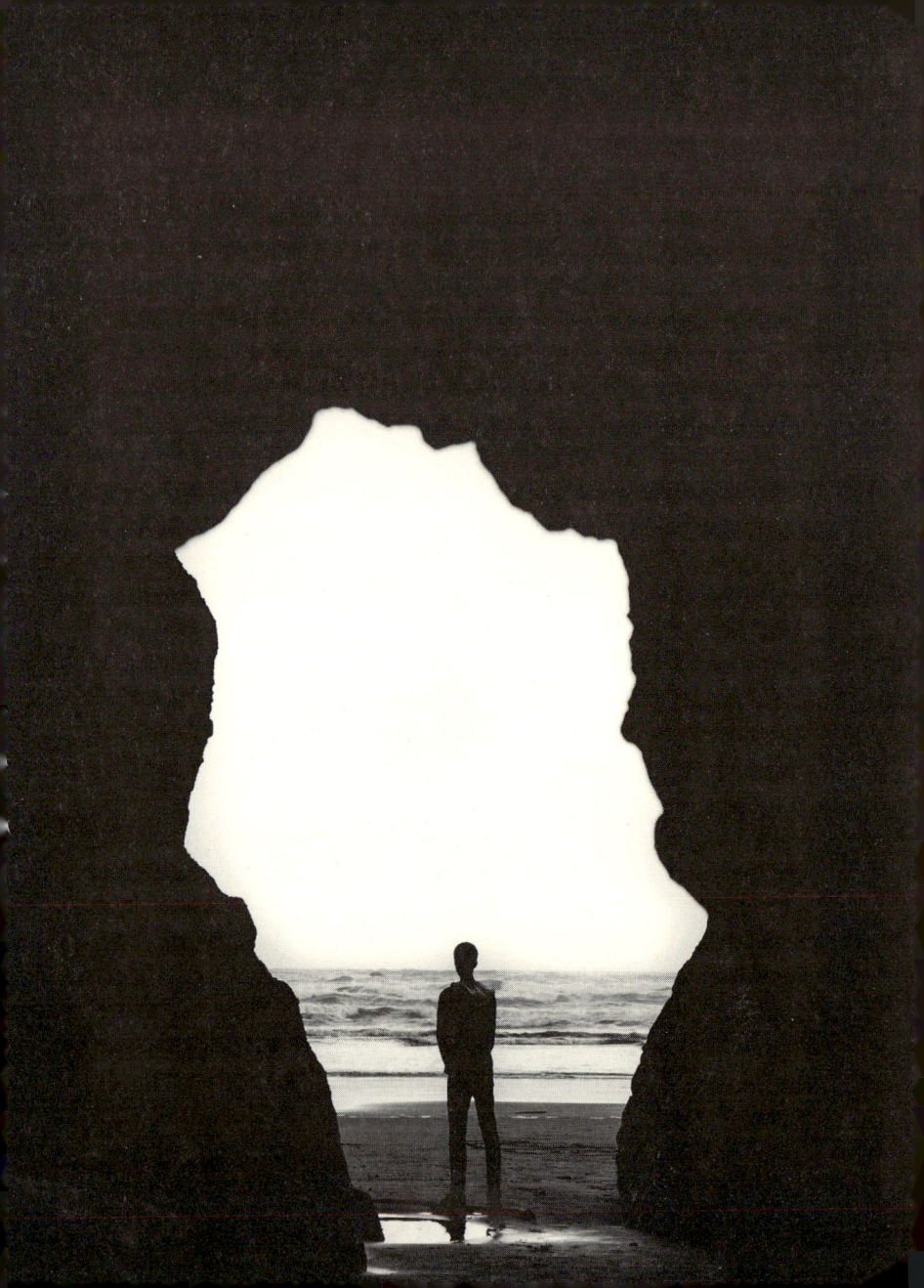

INTRODUCTION

Amrita Tripathi

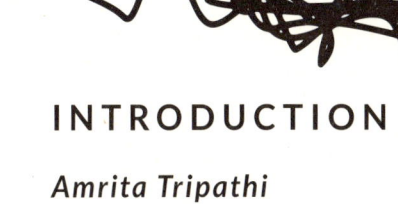

The idea behind the Mindscape series, which kicked off with the title *Real Stories of Living with Depression*, was to share stories of lived experiences that might resonate with others, and centre the narrative of mental health and mental illness firmly in India — that is, to look at stories, shared experiences and 'expert' views, with an India lens. We want to learn how to talk about mental health and mental disorders, about stress and emotional triggers, about complicated and often-life-altering diagnoses in a less complicated way.

We want to share stories and learnings and talk to experts, all the while understanding that there is an increasing push to focus on the psycho-social aspect of mental illness, that there is no one-size-fits-all model of diagnosis and care, and that the narrative needs to be centred around and led by those of us living with a given condition or diagnosis, who are as much the experts on their lives, as the psychologists and psychiatrists who have made it their life's work.

Young
MENTAL HEALTH

We want to do this in a way that is accessible and conversational, not overwhelming the reader with technical jargon. We also want this book to provide an entry point for the layperson interested in mental health, focusing on Young Mental Health, and providing a fairly structured narrative, with links for additional reading and more resources at the end.

So how do we go about this admittedly daunting challenge?

First, by facing the facts.

You can't start doing any research on mental health in India without bumping into startling, even painful statistics — the disease burden, lack of resources, and shockingly low numbers of trained professionals.

Speaking to Child and Adolescent Mental Health experts like Dr Amit Sen and co-author, psychologist and psychotherapist Meera Haran Alva, and looking at the available literature on the field of Young Mental Health, major topics that come up include:

- Depression, Anxiety and Stress (DAS)
- Bullying
- Learning and Behavioural Issues
- Suicidal Ideation
- Self-Harm
- Body Image and Eating Disorders

The need for intervention couldn't be more critical. And yet, many of us don't even know how to begin to have conversations before a situation hits crisis mode.

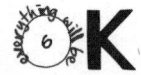

That's what this book is here for.

WHAT DO WE MEAN BY 'YOUNG MENTAL HEALTH'?

Young Mental Health usually covers child and adolescent mental health.

For the purpose of this book, we'll be focusing on adolescents and young adults, relying on those with lived experiences, who look back on their journeys through childhood and adolescence, even young adulthood. We can use their stories, their words to learn what to look out for — and even — how to talk about some difficult topics.

We are covering major issues that arise in the field of Young Mental Health in the traditional sense, via interviews with mental health experts and through the experience of co-author, psychologist and psychotherapist Meera Haran Alva, who has worked as a school psychologist and in independent practice for more than a decade and a half.

As someone who has suffered (needlessly and pointlessly, I may add) from disordered eating and self-harm over the years, as well as someone who has (needlessly and pointlessly) suffered from the shame of these 'aberrant' behaviours and thoughts, and who despite the adolescent cynicism (and let's admit it, the anger) could have used a hug or some sense of tribe or community back in the day, or even some reassurance that things were going to be okay ... let me just say now to each of you, to any young folks reading this, and to each of our younger selves: We're going to be okay. We can do this.

Young
MENTAL HEALTH

Together, we can learn or unlearn, as the need arises.

After all, we're not born knowing how to talk about bullying, or relationship stress, or anxiety, or pressure. But we can learn how to recognise the signs that can be a cause for concern. We can learn to acknowledge that suicide is the leading cause of death in the age group of 15–29 years[2] — that's the first step in learning how to talk about the heart-breaking reality. We need to mainstream these conversations — together.

As for each of you, dear readers, take this at your own pace. Also, please be aware that there are trained counsellors and helplines operational in this country at any time that you feel you want to reach out. We have included a list at the end of this book and a reference link[3]. If you are sharing from this book or talking to others, please be mindful of the best practice guidelines — with complicated issues like suicide, it is vital and even *life-saving* for us to follow protocols. **Always let people know that help is available.**

...

If you or anyone you know feels suicidal; or is talking about 'ending it all', please reach out to a trained professional for help. Know that you are not alone.
Some contact information and India-based helplines are here; more can be found at: http://www.healthcollective.in/suicide-prevention-helplines/.
Please note that these are third-party helplines
(verified as functional at the time of writing this book).

- Sneha India: 044-2464 0050/044-2464 0060 (24×7)
- Vandrevala Foundation: 18602662345 (24×7)
- iCall (TISS): 022-25521111 (Monday to Saturday, 8 am to 10 pm)

LEGAL DISCLAIMER: The Health Collective is not in the business of nor intends to provide counselling service. The professionals, the website of the professionals and helpline numbers listed on The Health Collective or in this book are not employed, associated or endorsed by The Health Collective. The professionals and the organisations behind the listed websites and helpline numbers, on The Health Collective website or reproduced in this book, are independent third-parties and there is no relationship of principal-agent, employer-employee, partnership of any nature with The Health Collective. The Health Collective, the publishers of this book and the authors do not make any recommendation or guarantee service or quality of any professional or helpline number or website listed herein. The Health Collective does not make any representations, warranties or guarantees as to, and is in no manner responsible for, the services provided by the professionals or their websites or the helpline services. The stories and comics set out by The Health Collective are intended purely for reference purposes. Advice or stories set out herein are by no means intended to malign or defame any person, organisation, caste or community. Advice or stories set out herein are views of the concerned authors only, The Health Collective does not claim copyright or endorse or recommend or represent on veracity of the advice contained in the articles or stories (including the comics) on this website or reproduced in this book. Additionally, the articles and stories set out herein should not in any manner be considered as a substitute for professional help. All experiences are personal, hence advice and suggestions contained in the articles and stories may not apply to a reader's specific facts or situations, and it is recommended that professional help is sought for such matters. The Health Collective, the publishers and authors disclaim all liability of all nature arising out of reliance placed on the advice set out in the stories or arising out of meetings with professionals or calls with the professionals or helpline numbers mentioned on the website of The Health Collective or in this book.

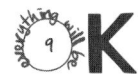

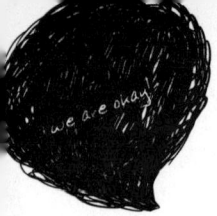

ABOUT THIS BOOK

PART 1 features interviews, lived experience, studies, comics and conversations with young adults who take a look back at their own journeys that they want to share. We have built on our work as The Health Collective website (www.healthcollective.in), which features some 300 stories as of early 2020, including stories of lived experiences, original reportage, expert columns and original artwork. We are very grateful to contributors who agreed to share more, dig even deeper and excavate some of their most vulnerable memories, in the hopes that their stories would resonate with others.

PART 2 of this book includes some important information and practical tips by Meera Haran Alva, who draws on her experience as a school psychologist and family therapist to share a clinical-based approach on what to look out for, what therapies are available for various conditions and a 'toolbox' that applies for each, including approaches that have worked. We also feature some moving first person stories and comics, as well as interviews with key stakeholders that should help round out our understanding of some critical issues.

We'll also share more information on:

- Depression, Anxiety and Stress (often called DAS, and believed to be one of the key areas in the field of Young Mental Health)
  - Pressure (academic pressure, relationship stress, parental pressure)
  - Coping Strategies for Bullying
  - Suicidal Ideation (and young suicide)
  - Self-Harm, Eating Disorders, Body Image Disorder
  - Parental To Do's and (ideally) Not Do's
  - When to Reach out for Professional Help

For those of you looking for specific information, the table of contents will guide you — we have interviews, lived experiences, anecdotes in the first half, as well as illustrations and comics, and a more in-depth look at certain conditions as well as exercises meant for parents in the second half.

Make your notes, share your feedback, and always get a second opinion if you can.

Most of us need to stop internalising the sense of shame or failure of 'letting someone down', of 'meddling where we're not wanted'. Together, we can learn to remove our egos or self-consciousness from the equation, whether as siblings, parents, friends, and just ask each other: *Are you doing okay? Do you want to talk? If not to me, can I get you someone else to talk to?*

Thanks to Devanik Saha, who went through and compiled several key India-based studies on *Young Mental Health*, which helped inform this work. Thanks also to Pattie Gonsalves of Sangath for sharing a few additional studies, and as always to the experts and interviewees, The Health Collective team and tribe of well-wishers. We are indebted to all of you, but solely responsible for anything missing or any oversight, and are striving to be ever-more inclusive, going forward.

Also be assured that this is meant to be a conversational, even gentle book, not a long lecture with a lot of '*You Should*' or '*Why Haven't You*' or '*How Could You*' or anything of the sort. Feel free to pick it up, put it down ... pick it up again. Lend it around.

And stay well.

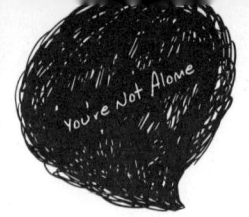

MOVING IN THE RIGHT DIRECTION
Meera Haran Alva

Over the past 17 years of my psychotherapy practice, I have witnessed a significant shift in how mental health is viewed in a less stigmatising way.

This is in the context of the urban, economically more affluent sections of India. There seems to be a marked difference in how Indians, especially from the younger strata, are open to seeking therapy. I have seen a huge spike in the number of referrals I have received over the past few years and I am often at a loss when it comes to referring them to another professional.

There is a huge dearth of mental health professionals in the country with an estimated number of only 0.047 trained psychologists per 1,00,000 people who are in need of mental health care[4]. The Mental Health Care Act 2017, a bill that replaced the older Act of 1987, compels the state to have a mental health programme to respond to the growing need for trained mental health professionals to bridge this gap in treatment.

I am excited about the new discourses and conversations happening around mental health in the print media, on social media, television and in the movies as this has had a very positive impact on how we talk about mental health in our homes, schools, work spaces and communities. This movement toward acceptance of mental health-related issues is the need of the hour and as a practitioner I feel the urgency to advocate for it.

In the more privileged, urban Indian schools there are waves of positive systemic changes with principals and other leaders in the school talking about the need for inclusion and are implementing it by setting up learning support services and programmes for children with disabilities. I see this as being extremely significant from a philosophical point of view — to practice and believe in inclusion is to embrace and accept children with all their differences and unique facets. This is most critical to their sense of well-being and holistic development.

On the other hand, we are also faced with the alarming reality of the 80 per cent of children in rural India without provisions for special schools or for the eight million children who are out of school, marginalised, because of factors such as poverty, gender, disability and caste[5]. These stark differences are overwhelming to grapple with knowing how crucial it is for every child to have their fundamental right to education and their developmental needs fulfilled. The hope is to see that school systems take accountability and responsibility to address these differing needs of children and adolescents and not the other way around where they are expected to make do and 'fit in' with what the school has to offer.

The implementation of the psycho-education based programmes as an integral part of the school curriculum is a great move in educating children about mental health. These programmes are called PSD (psycho-social development) or PSE (psycho-social education) lessons that are taught by the school counsellor or psychology teacher on a weekly basis. These lessons lend opportunities to teach and discuss life skills and topics that are connected to the child's emotional and psychological well-being.

Children and teenagers of today seem more aware about psychological and mental health-related issues as a result of these programmes. It has become okay to say that you are depressed and 'trendy' to see a therapist. While I have my concerns about 'it being cool' as a motive to see me, what is heartening is the openness and acceptability of having conversations about it. It is no longer something to be whispered about.

According to a study[6] done by the Department of Psychiatry, National Institute of Mental Health and Neurosciences (NIMHANS, Bangalore) in 2010, life skills education integrated into the school mental health programmes using available resources of schools and teachers is seen as an effective way of empowering adolescents.

While these programmes are helping adolescents with their life skills development, there still remains a great concern among mental health professionals in India about the connection between heightened expectations of educational success and a rise of mental health problems among young people[7].

To address these rising pressures on school students, which in some cases are leading to suicides, the Indian government has made counselling centres led by clinical psychologists as mandatory in government and private schools. These also include CBSE and ICSE schools in India. This has made counselling more accessible to children and families in a school setting.

Part of my motivation to push to do better and work to improve the state of child and adolescent mental health services in India dates back to my internship during the 2nd year of my masters' programme in clinical psychology. My internship at the famous All India Medical Hospital turned out to be very disillusioning, not least because of the lack of sensitivity and empathy — the 'patients' who came in left sometimes perhaps more distraught than before. I still remember a mother who was very anxious, waiting to receive the result of an IQ assessment of her child sitting across the table from a psychologist, who was surrounded by awkward PG students such as myself. The psychologist without much affect declared to her, '*Aapka bacha kudrathi se aisa hai* (Your child is like this by nature).' She continued with utter apathy about the child having a low IQ, and 'that is how it is'. I felt all sorts of anger that day and indeed through the year.

Fast forward 17 years, and I am slightly more optimistic about the state of affairs in urban India, but a lot of work needs to be done.

I have since then worked in schools in Delhi, Mumbai and Bangalore gaining insights into the interesting dynamics and workings of schools and families in the urban Indian context. The great thing about working in a school is that children and adolescents are able to access mental health services more easily as there is no additional fee that the parents need to pay and all that the children require to avail the service is parental consent. At times the child would use the excuse of academic stress as a pretext to schedule a session with me and use this time to work on their self, family and peer issues.

In my private practice, I tend to see children and families when problems have escalated to a great degree. This is my biggest concern. Parents and teachers wait too long before noticing that a child needs help. This denial and delay results in the neglect of the child's well-being. I am also aware that in India, we do not have as many professionals in the system in comparison to the need for mental health services.

Families in crisis are also often at a loss to know whom they need to see when their situation escalates. Unfortunately, there is an absence of licensing associations in India to help identify or offer a database of verified practitioners. Hence there are individuals who are practicing unethically, affecting those who are vulnerable and at risk. For this, it is helpful to check the credentials of the therapists you choose. Ensure that they have the qualifications and training necessary to be psychotherapists or clinical psychologists.

WHO IS A PSYCHOLOGIST?

A professional who has a postgraduate degree in psychology. They are trained to do counselling, psychological testing and research. They need additional training to practise psychotherapy.

WHO IS A CLINICAL PSYCHOLOGIST?

A professional who has an MPhil or doctoral degree in clinical psychology. They are trained to do psychological testing for diagnostic and assessment purposes. They are also trained in specific models of therapy to address mental health issues.

WHO IS A PSYCHOTHERAPIST?

A professional who has a postgraduate degree in psychotherapy. Psychotherapy can be long term, insight-based talking. Psychotherapists can do individual therapy, couples therapy or child and family therapy depending on their training.

WHO IS A COUNSELLOR?

A professional who goes through a shorter formal training in counselling. Their work may be more short term, supportive and issue-based talking.

WHO IS A PSYCHIATRIST?

A professional who is a medical doctor who has specialised in psychiatry. They

can prescribe medication for and diagnose mental illnesses. They do not practice psychotherapy, as this is not a part of their medical education.

You can find more information on where to seek help in publicly available databases like **www.healthcollective.in/contact**, which link to crowd-sourced materials, including the widely shared iCall document.

It's important to equip ourselves with as much knowledge as we can on what is a complicated subject, but please do not attempt to self-diagnose or diagnose anyone without help from those with the right professional expertise.

WHAT TO EXPECT IN THIS BOOK

In Part 2 of this book, I have a handbook for parents, where you will find information regarding:

- Who is a 'normal' child?
- What is a family?
- Why is it helpful to have a systemic perspective with respect to your child's well-being?
- What is child and adolescent therapy? What can you expect?
- How do you make a decision about the need for therapy?
- What do you look out for when you are concerned if your child may be depressed or anxious? (Please note that this is just a checklist and is not meant for formal diagnosis. Only a psychiatrist can diagnose and prescribe medication.)
- What can you do if your child is diagnosed with depression or anxiety?
- Tools that can help you engage with as a family, which can be therapeutic when you or your child feels anxious or depressed. (Please note: This is not a substitute for therapy, these are more complementary in nature, consider them to be 'holding' techniques.)
- Information about child sexual abuse: Warning signs and what to do if your

child tells you about abuse.

When I work with children and their parents I feel their pain and concern. As a parent myself, I understand the challenges of parenting. No matter what you may know and understand you are never fully prepared for it. I have learnt that it is human, helpful and absolutely OKAY to reach out to seek support from friends, family and professionals. I am afraid our families alone are not adequate and enough of a support system to rely on. There is no shame in seeking psychotherapy services, it is not a reflection on your abilities or skills as a parent or that there is something wrong with your child.

Like any parent, I worry about my children and feel protective of them in light of what they might be exposed to with what's happening in the world — discrimination based on gender, sexuality, religion, race, etc. I want to bring love, hope and strength to them and to all the children and families I work with.

I feel gratitude towards all my clients who have worked with me and from whom I have learned so much. We hope that this book will provide the readers with helpful information on Young Mental Health and the courage to seek help and support. As a parent of a teen and a tween, I understand how challenging parenting can be and I couldn't have done it so far without the support I have received from my family, friends, school and other professional resources. I believe it is true that it takes a village to raise a child but more importantly a village where all the members jointly understand the needs of the child and love the child unconditionally.

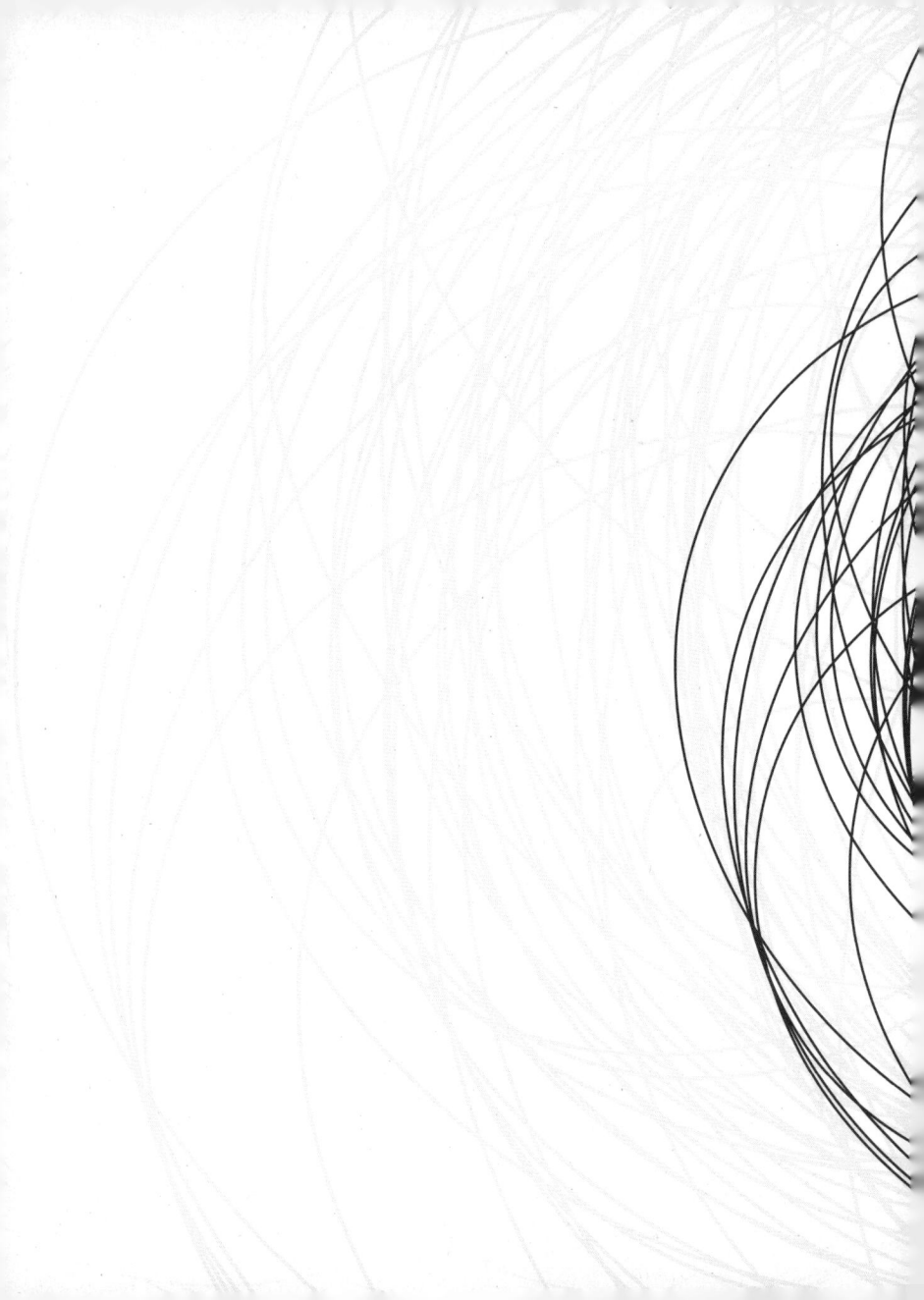

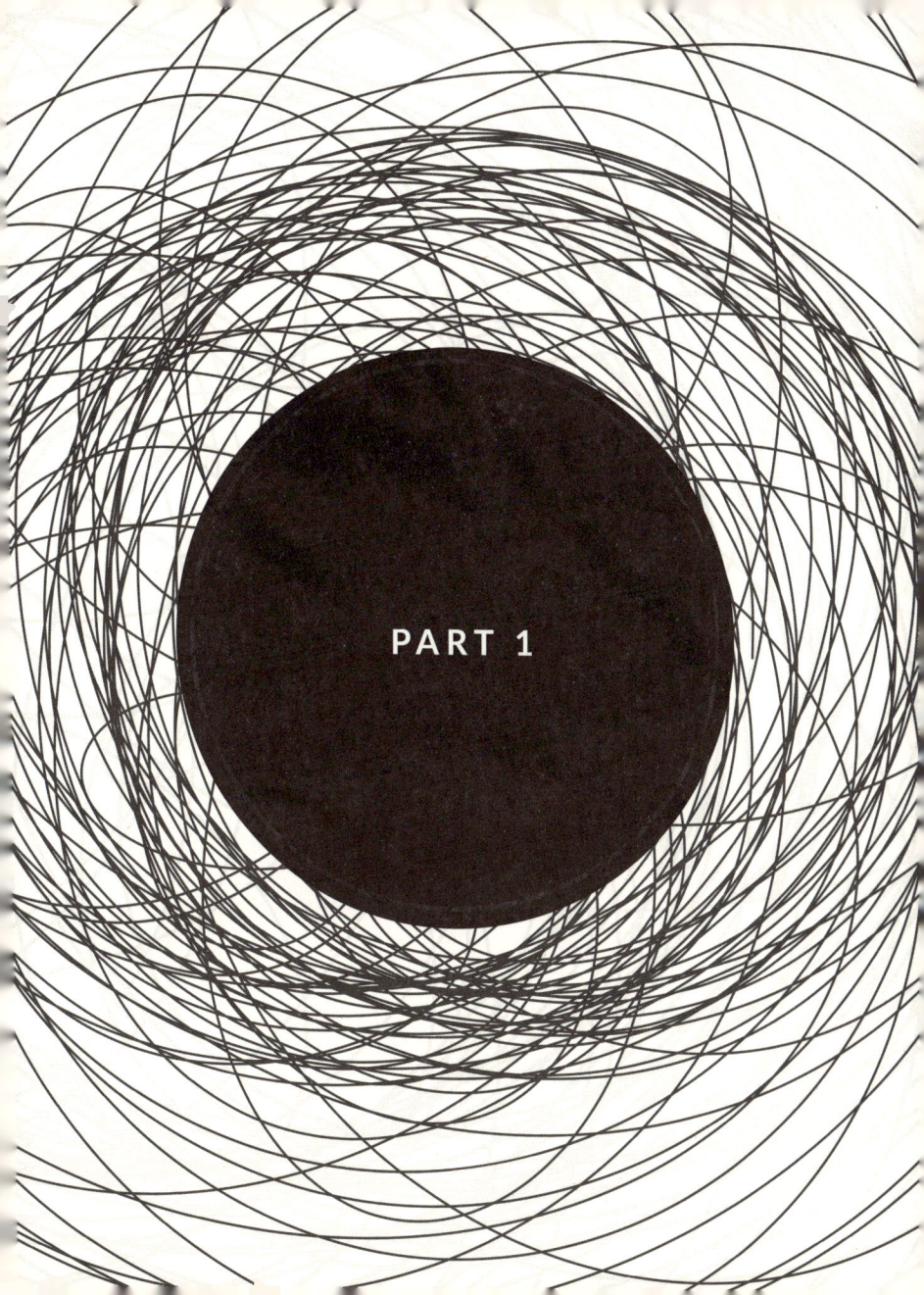

PART 1

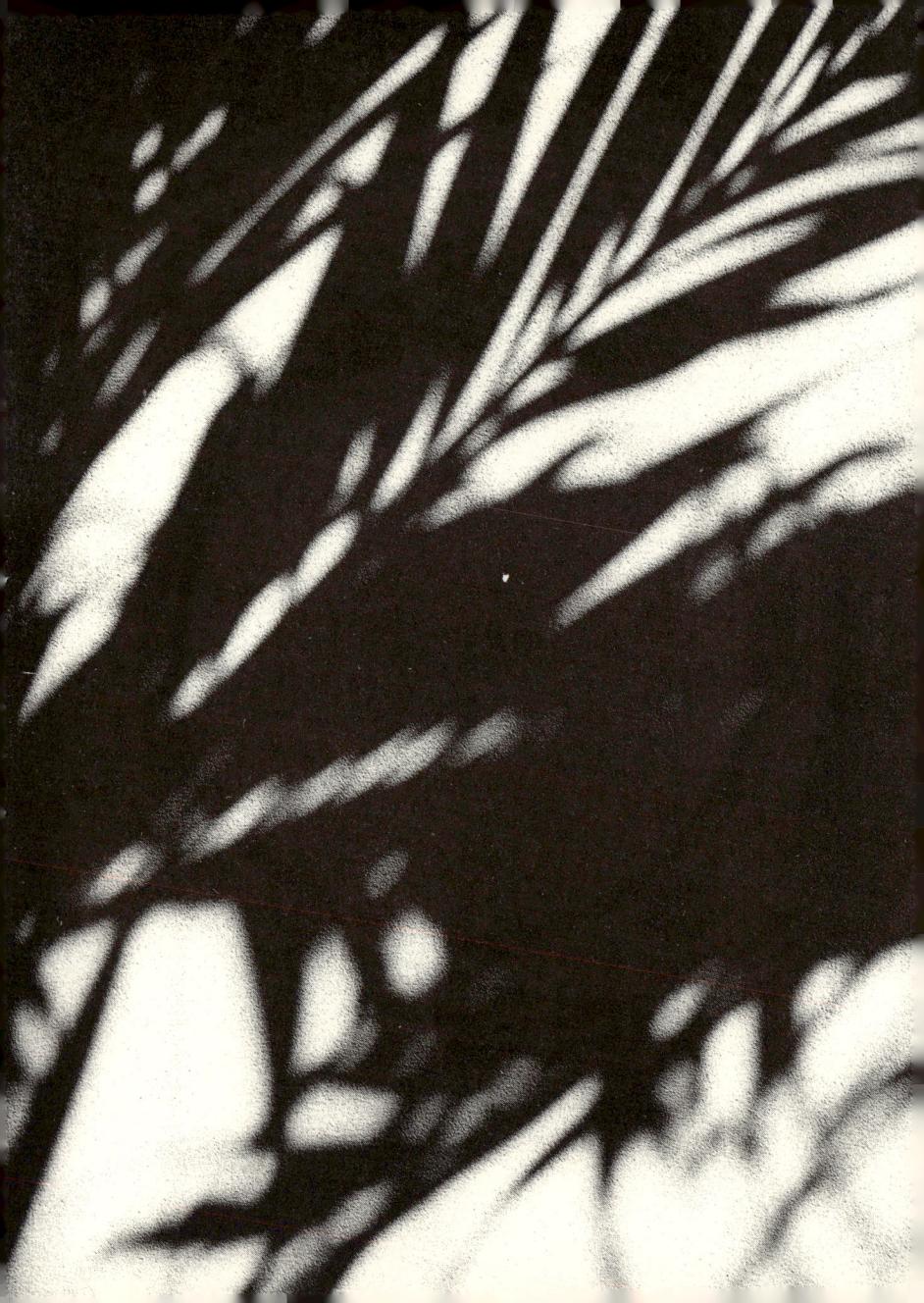

Chapter 1
THE CONTEXT: WHY YOUNG MENTAL HEALTH MATTERS

Let's take a slightly closer look at why it's important to face the facts, before we dive straight in. Mental health and mental illness affect all of us, of whatever age. In India, the fact of the matter is, not enough of us are getting the help we need. And that includes Young India.

...

- Mental health issues are estimated to affect 150 million Indians[8]
- Less than 30 million Indians are seeking care[9]
- Suicide is the leading cause of death for Indians in the age group of 15– 39 years[10]

As NIMHANS director Professor B.N. Gangadhar's introduction to the landmark National Mental Health Survey (NMHS) 2015–16 commissioned by the Ministry of Health and Family Welfare writes:

'The results from the NMHS point to the huge burden of mental health problems: while, nearly 150 million Indians need mental health care services, less than 30 million are seeking care; the mental health systems assessment indicate not just a lack of public health strategy but also several under-performing components.'[11]

WHAT ABOUT YOUNG INDIA?

The National Mental Health Survey mentions a pilot study that examined the 'mental morbidity' of adolescents (from the ages of 13–17) in four of the 12 states covered by the survey. It goes on to say, 'The overall prevalence of any mental morbidity was 7.3% with a similar distribution between males and females (M: 7.5%; F: 7.1%) ... Interestingly, the problem in urban metro regions was higher as compared to rural and urban non-metro areas (13.5% vs. 6.9% and 4.3% respectively).'[12]

An article in *BMC Psychology* (by R. Parikh et al) notes that India is home to more than 250 million adolescents, about one-fifth of the world's adolescents, going on to say ... 'studies conducted among school-going adolescents in urban India indicate that at least one in five adolescents endure high stress levels in their daily lives [9–13].'[13]

Let that sink in: One in five adolescents is dealing with high stress daily. While we often think of this age group and dismiss the stress as 'exam stress' or 'nothing out of the ordinary, as this is a difficult age', that doesn't tell the whole story.

This study, conducted via 22 focus groups, focusing on eight Delhi government-run high schools and a private school, as well as seven high schools in Goa, found that the most common stressors for the students, aged 11–17 years, was:

- Academic Pressure
- Stress from Negotiating Autonomy (limited personal freedoms, including parental influences and peer pressure)
- Safety (including threatened violence, physical sexual harassment, bullying, physical punishment, domestic violence)

And then there are socio-economic factors at play, which need to also be taken into account. Quoting from the same study: 'Additionally, younger adolescents in Delhi highlighted poverty and consequent hopelessness as stressors.'[14]

Things are even more dire than that if you look at the prevalence of suicidal ideation and suicide.

As an article[15] written by youth advocate, Mohit Dhingra, for The Health Collective on the occasion of World Mental Health Day 2019 says, 'Statistics don't usually justify the on-ground scenarios and the complexity of an issue but here are some anyway. India saw a jump in the number of suicides to a total of 2,30,314, as submitted by *The Lancet Public Health*, 2018.'[16] For the age groups of 15–39 years, suicide was found to be the most common cause of death. India makes up for nearly 37 per cent of global female suicide deaths and 25 per cent of global male suicide deaths.[17]

Who do we refer people to? We have listed a few helplines in the Introduction and you'll find more on our website (ww.healthcollective.in/suicide-prevention-helplines). But the fact of the matter is we also simply don't have enough trained mental health experts in India — the number is a fraction of what it should be.

Young
MENTAL HEALTH

To quote from the author of *How To Travel Light: My Memories of Madness and Melancholia*, Shreevatsa Nevatia's article in *HuffPost India*, 'On 9 February, Anupriya Patel, (then) Minister of State for Health and Family Welfare, told the Lok Sabha that India had only 3,827 registered psychiatrists. It needed at least 13,500. In comparison, the United States had about 28,000 psychiatrists in 2017. Patel also told Parliament that India required 20,250 clinical psychologists, but had only 898.'[18]

While there is a clear need for more trained mental health experts, that treatment or care gap isn't going to magically vanish overnight. Ideally, we will need to find that happy middle ground where enough of us laypersons equip ourselves with enough knowledge to know when someone needs professional help and, crucially, where to find access to that help. What each one of us can sign on for is to acquire more tools to equip ourselves with awareness, self-awareness, empathy, and even empathetic listening.

Each of us has a role to play in a community or society or family and each of us can learn to tackle stigma by choosing that it ends with us. If you or I can drop our hesitation and fear or terror (often born of ignorance) about some very common conditions, then maybe you and I can become better allies on the ground for those who need us.

'Is this really my problem?' Some of you might be asking.

Well, yes, probably so. Given all the statistics, it's very unlikely that you and I can afford to remain oblivious even if we choose to. But don't think only of mental illness or disorders — mental health affects each and every one of us, as experts like Dr Vikram Patel and Dr Amit Sen, and several youth mental health advocates teach us.

There is increasingly a call to see mental health issues in the socio-cultural contexts in which they arise — Paras Sharma of The Alternative Story shares with us that he feels, 'definitely there is fatigue, burn-out, isolation... worry, anxiety, lack of meaning, lack of fulfilment, which are all experiences which are nearly universal for young people right now.' In his interview, we will learn more on how to look at mental health through an intersectional, feminist and existential lens.

Mental disorders too affect almost every family or friends' circle, if you start thinking about this even anecdotally. The root causes of what can grow into more serious conditions begins in childhood, so it's perhaps fitting that we look at the foundation of our mental health, and try to unravel some of the complicated webs that can begin with emotional distress and lead to trauma and other severe repercussions.

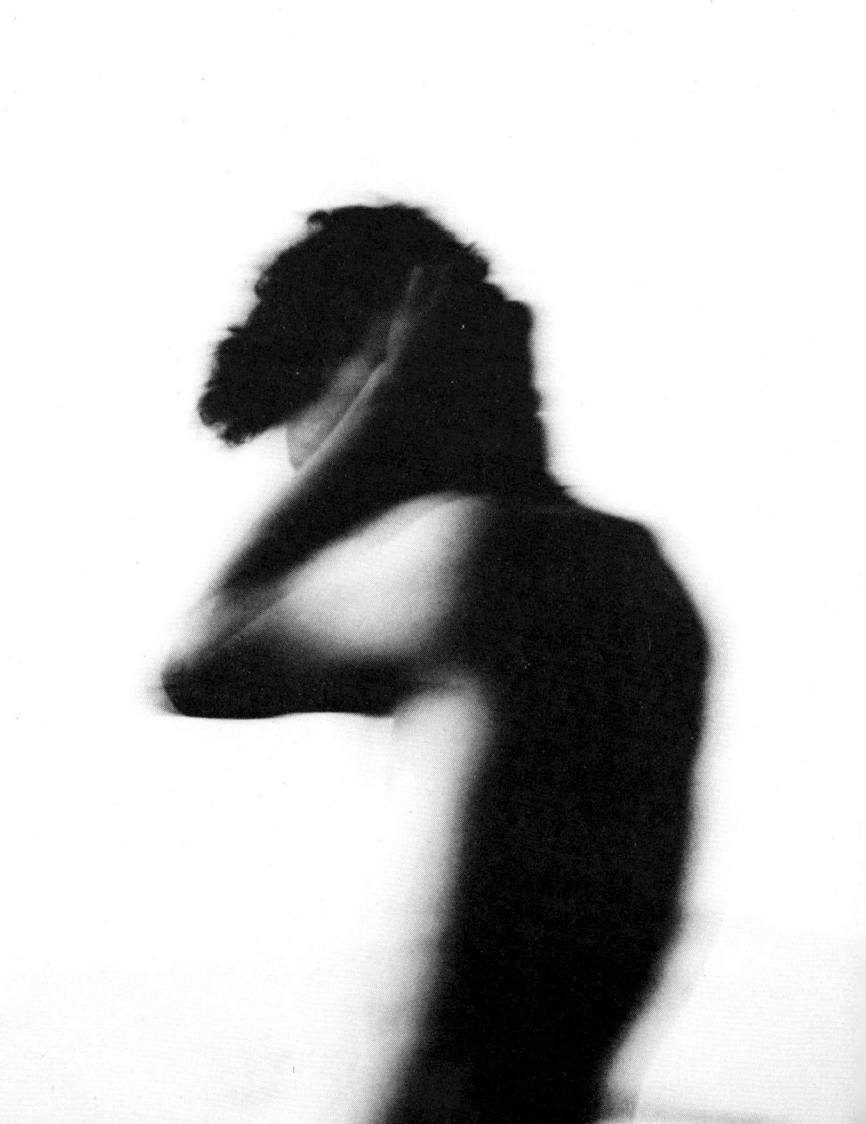

Chapter 2
WHAT'S STRESSING OUT INDIA'S KIDS?

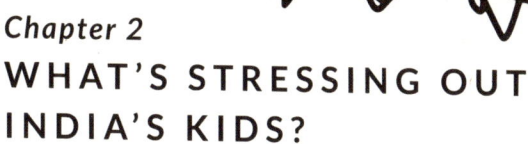

Dr Amit Sen is a well-known Delhi-based child and adolescent psychiatrist with three decades of experience in psychiatry. He has worked predominantly with children and adolescents, he shares, for 25 of the last 31 years. He, along with Dr Shelja Sen and Dr Kavita Arora, set up the centre, Children First, in Delhi almost a decade ago, and has seen close to 9,000 registrations in that period of time. Referrals to Children First come in not just from the National Capital Region, but also cities like Bareilly, Kanpur, Lucknow, Jaipur, Jalandhar, Amritsar, Srinagar and even smaller towns.

This chapter stems from interviews conducted in December 2017 and September 2019, where Dr Sen not only highlights some of the most common stressors for children and adolescents in India, but also traces the trajectory of awareness in India in the past several years.

Young MENTAL HEALTH

AMRITA: We're in conversation today with senior psychiatrist Dr Amit Sen who will take us through some of the most common stressors when it comes to child and adolescent mental health.

DR AMIT SEN: I think in India, one stressor that runs across all of childhood and adolescence is academics — education or the way education is viewed in our country. Schooling starts very early and a lot of our kids are not ready neuro-developmentally to engage with it in the way they are expected to by schools, by teachers, parents.

A lot of these kids spend large amounts of their time trying to learn things, which perhaps they're not ready for; at the expense of play time, building bonds, relationships, just being free and having fun. The pressure and expectations keep rising as kids go from Nursery, KG to primary school. The pressure starts very early, and even when a three-year-old is not able to do what they are expected to by a teacher, alarm bells start ringing. Parents start worrying, and usually start by disciplining or scolding the child. At the end of it, they might really begin to worry about the future of their children and take them to specialists and so on.

The system is to blame. In our country, we start with academic learning way too early, and a large part of expectations is driven by rote-learning. There is hardly any flexibility and we see this right across primary school; as they get into secondary, middle and senior school, the expectations get higher. The manifestations of that pressure are not seen so much in primary school, though sometimes they are. We do sometimes see children for anxiety and behaviour disturbances only due to academic pressure in primary school. But more often than not, they keep piling up and it's like a dam bursting when they reach adolescence. That's when you begin to see depression and anxiety and a range of other issues, like substance misuse, so-called oppositional defiant disordered behaviours. So it's a relentless and eroding, oppressive system that we put our children through.

AMRITA: Something else you've said you can track from childhood on is relationships, and stress due to relationships.

DR AMIT SEN: Yes, of course. Relationships no doubt are key and the cornerstone of emotional and social development of any child. Again, because of some of the other demands which are placed on children, sometimes we see the parent–child relationship begins to be affected very early, in primary school.

The time that parents might have had to just be with their kids or play with their kids or be without pressure and anxiety is simply diminishing. As they grow up, other kinds of relationships become important, peer relationships, relationships through social media of various kinds. And those become extremely complicated and warped at times.

Although social media is a great thing, you find that for young people it becomes central in their lives. How many thumbs up they've got, how many likes they've got, what kind of persona they are able to project, who is bullying whom on social media, who is getting ostracised and so on. A large part of their waking hours are being spent just engaging with that. And those relationships are so complex.
Adults, because we have so little knowledge about this whole dynamic of the social media world, are hardly able to guide them; adults come down very heavily, take

away gadgets of young people or admonish them. We have to accept that young people know so much more, have such a mastery over it that we can't stop them from getting into it unless we come on the same side and try and understand it.

AMRITA: Could you take us through maybe two or three things you wish all parents would know when it comes to this age group?

DR AMIT SEN: One of the things I often find parents do is that believe once children have become teenagers, they have grown up and don't need parental supervision anymore. For instance, we see this when we do parenting workshops in schools. When we do it in junior school, there's a very impressive turnout, but when we do it in senior or middle school we hardly have any parents turn up. It's like they've given up on their kids or they don't think it's important anymore, this whole business of parenting, building relationships, guiding them through their teenage years as they grow into adults.

And that is one of the most vulnerable periods, and I don't think parents give it that importance. They don't invest in it. And sometimes because kids show some independence and some rebellion perhaps, and don't want parents to get into their personal or social spaces, they back off. Again, if you look at the trajectory of parents and their careers, for instance, when children become teenagers, they're in their mid-40s or close to 50 perhaps, and that's also the time when their careers are taking off, you know, there are big decisions to be made for the family, their own parents are getting older and so on. So for various reasons, I think they tend to disengage from young teenaged children, and that can often lead these kids astray, for want of a better word. Because there are so many opportunities now, it's not just the neighbourhood, it's the big wide social media world, that can be so exploitative.

So if you do not — or are not able to — get into your young person's world, or engage them in conversations such as, 'What do relationships mean?' and 'What does being successful mean to you?', or 'What does being good or bad mean to you?', they might not be able to pick these concepts up as easily. These are things we take for granted. People believe children will intuitively pick it up or understand as soon as parents label them. But that's not the case, because the definitions of things have changed, they've changed and we have to have a conversation about it. And understand from their perspective and then help them, perhaps through questions or reflections to help them make good choices.

You can't say that 'I've spent so much time with children in primary school they should automatically behave well with me as adolescents.' It doesn't work like that! Because their influences are varied and they're vast and different from how they were 20 years ago. So they will bring a lot from school, from peers, from social media back into their homes, into relationships with their parents and as parents we need to understand where they are coming from.

Sometimes young people by nature will put up a facade not to reveal a lot of the turmoil they are going through. They want to look grown up, they want to look confident. So even if they have a lot of conflicts or turbulence inside, they're unlikely to reveal to someone who doesn't have that time to listen. So you have to build that relationship of trust, of deep listening, that non-judgemental listening where you can encourage your kids to open up perhaps, and only then will you know a little bit of their world!

...

In this section, you'll find excerpts of an interview with Dr Sen from September 2019. (Trigger warning: Self-harm, suicidal ideation, trauma, abuse, eating disorders)

AMRITA: Given your 31 years (of work as a psychiatrist), I do want to ask if you have noticed a change of awareness of Young Mental Health issues, with families and schools? You would have seen a 'pre'- era when, for example, people didn't know you could reach out for help with certain things.

DR AMIT SEN: Absolutely. When I first started training in psychiatry, I trained in NIMHANS (The National Institute of Mental Health and Neurosciences), which had a dedicated child and adolescent psychiatry unit. They used to get referrals from across the country. Those referrals would be of children who were clearly outside the norm, in terms of development or behaviours. They would come only when things would really get out of hand, or out of control. They would be tertiary care referrals. Once I started working in the private sector, about 15–16 years ago, there was this notion that a stand-alone child and adolescent service is not going to run, because the demand is not as much. We were told by our senior colleagues, 'Don't put all your eggs in one basket, as it's probably not going to work.' We'd just returned from England — it was then Shelja (Dr Shelja Sen) and I — and we said, 'No, this is what we want to do and the need is there and we're not quite aware of it yet.'

A year prior to that, I had gone to different parts of the country to do a kind of survey of services of what's required, and it seemed to me the need was much more than was apparent. It took a year or two to pick up, but soon we were inundated with referrals. However, the pattern was families would bring their children to us only when the situation was dire and again it was completely out of control.
Also, with developmental disorders like autism, they would come to us much later in the chronological years, many would come during adolescence or when they were eight or 10 years old, by which time a lot would have happened in their lives, in terms of how they were treated. Families would only bring their children to us when they realised nothing is changing.

Many times, when children don't speak at the right time or don't do things as they're supposed to when they're younger, many people in the family will say, '*Oh theek ho jayega*', or 'My child also spoke at five, or I spoke at five ... why do you worry?' And things like that. And many times, paediatricians would give the same kind of messages. The parents would end up waiting/delaying and coming in for a referral much later in the developmental years, which is not optimal.

Now, say with autism, the majority of the kids who come to us are between the ages of two to four — which means the awareness has grown of the possibility of this being something that needs urgent and early attention and intervention. And the stigma has gone down too, so people much more readily actually access us. Now the referrals again from paediatricians, sometimes from adult psychiatrists and from schools, have started coming much earlier. Sometimes parents will research about us on the net and make a self-referral. I think the number of referrals that come to us has increased exponentially. There is a cluster of developmental difficulties like autism, ADHD, other learning difficulties, sometimes maybe cerebral palsy — increasingly the age has become younger and younger. Now we have an infant development programme — our youngest one was five/six months old. So we have kids as young as that who come to us now.

Then you have the other spectrum like depression, anxiety, eating disorders, post-traumatic stress disorder, bipolar disorder, that you see in the older kids. And even there, the recognition of some of these changes in moods, behaviour patterns, relational difficulties, etc. have started raising worry and anxiety in the larger community (amongst parents, amongst teachers) much earlier than before.

So what has happened as a result, our service has not only grown at a rapid pace, but we are never ever able to fulfil all the need. We are constantly struggling with our waiting list, with the number of referrals we get. It keeps increasing, so we keep increasing the scope of our service, the capacity, we try to cut down the waiting time by doing many, many things, training another rung of specialists. If you look at the statistics, it's a deluge, it's like an epidemic of emotional, behavioural difficulties, and also developmental difficulties. When it came to autism — during the time I was training in psychiatry, doing my MD — the statistic was that there were two to three kids diagnosed with autism in 10,000. That rate has come down to one in 79, or

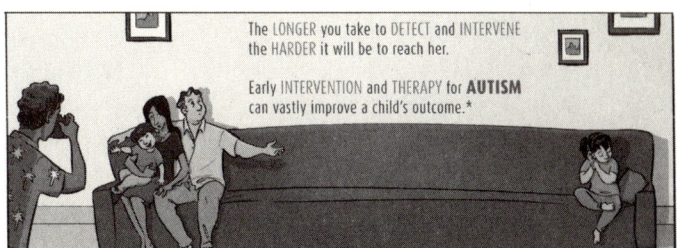

SOURCE: Journal of Autism and Developmental Disorders
Merryn John, Kishore Mohan | Health Collective

About the Artist: Kishore Mohan is a part-time dreamer, full-time artist, and impulsive wanderer, His cartoons and comic strips have been appearing in national dailies since 2008. Kishore has directed animation segments in the several movies and continues to work as a creative consultant and a pre-production/concept artist in the Indian film industry. You can find more on https://kishoremohan.blogspot.in

something. That's about 10/20 times the number. (That's a global figure.)

AMRITA: What do you see as some of the common issues that are present in a younger age group? And then from adolescence on, what are some of the most common things that you see?

DR AMIT SEN: If you look at the younger population, the reason they come to us are for two predominant things: one could be because they are not performing academically, from an early age. They're not learning their letters and numbers and so on, and the school is flagging it up, and parents get worried and come to us. This population will fall in the spectrum of neurodevelopmental disorders — including autism, ADHD, learning disabilities — and we see a lot of that.

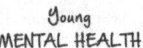
MENTAL HEALTH

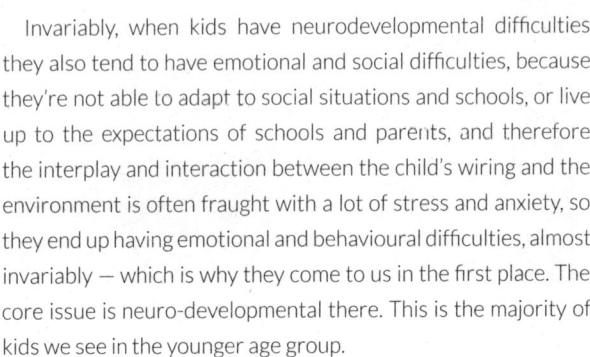

Invariably, when kids have neurodevelopmental difficulties, they also tend to have emotional and social difficulties, because they're not able to adapt to social situations and schools, or live up to the expectations of schools and parents, and therefore the interplay and interaction between the child's wiring and the environment is often fraught with a lot of stress and anxiety, so they end up having emotional and behavioural difficulties, almost invariably — which is why they come to us in the first place. The core issue is neuro-developmental there. This is the majority of kids we see in the younger age group.

We have an early intervention service here, specifically for children who are mostly within the autism spectrum, and those kids are getting younger and younger. We get kids who are one and a half, two, two and a half years old, who are coming for regular therapies. They could be very young, or they could be kids who are seven or eight, who are going to school and yet finding it a real struggle to keep up with the expectations and learning curve.

If you look at the older age group, then depression by far is the most common diagnosis or condition we see. But often it is not just depression, it is complicated by other things. Like a child who is otherwise bright, who has attention difficulties, who has not been identified as having ADHD very early, but later when they are 14 or 15, and facing academic demands when it comes to managing themselves, self-regulation, time management, organisational skills — what we call executive skills of the mind — they don't fall into place, and again they begin to get a lot of flak from the environment, for being lazy, for being a waster, for not using their potential and so on ... and that then precipitates a lot of anxiety and many times, depression.

So, although we see depression as the presenting feature, there could be undercurrents of other things. There could be changes in the family structure — broken families, reconstituted families, we see a lot of that. And both in the pre-pubertal age group and later, so often we see cases of bullying and social ostracisation, having a difficult time socially, break-ups in relationships and so on. The media has a big role to play now, because of how it plays out in their social lives, and how unless you get so many 'likes' you haven't made it in life, those kind of things affect teenagers so much.

We see an increasing number of eating disorders and also we see a lot of children who have gone through trauma in their lives. Some of the trauma that we see, again it might come up in therapy suddenly. A young person might remember what they went through when they were younger — it could be physical abuse, sexual abuse domestic violence etc ... and sometimes it's more subtle, it's emotional abuse and neglect because of so many different things — family situation or change of school — a wide range of things that could have affected them earlier in their lives.

We see a lot of kids who have gone through trauma of different kinds at different times.

Sometimes the trauma is because they've gotten into relationships early in their lives — 13 or 14 — and some of those relationships are very abusive or violent, and that can have deep impacts on their development, emotional development particularly.

Because we also work with a population such as street children and marginalised children, we see a lot of trauma from there too. And the effects of trauma are very devastating and deep.

The thing about trauma is that it doesn't often surface soon after the trauma occurs. It can surface many years afterwards, and it takes people by surprise. They're so confused, perplexed by the ferocity of what comes out then. That's something we often grapple with, along with families and schools and all of that.

In the older generation there is more awareness about personal boundaries and again, I think because some of the spaces socially are conducive for young people to open up and talk about these things, with the #MeToo movement and all that, many such things are coming up now in the young population. So we see in our clinics, many young people saying, '*I was raped in boarding school*', or '*I was abused by an older child*', or by a teacher.

AMRITA: Awareness is helpful if they can reach out but people have been talking about re-triggering (as well). If people haven't got access to help and are feeling re-triggered, do you have advice for them? Some people have been feeling that going through their social media feeds can be overwhelming or anxiety provoking. How does it impact them?

DR AMIT SEN: Of course, the thing is that the effect of such traumatic experiences at whatever stage in life will play out at some time or the other. It might play out at a conscious level when you begin to remember some of what's happened to you. Or it might happen in how you view the world and relationships and trust in people, your ability to form trusting, caring relationships or your ability to have a sense of self-worth — all those things get affected by trauma.

I do believe that the fact we are beginning to acknowledge this and provide or build safe spaces for young people to come out and talk about it, no doubt is going to be beneficial and healing for many who have gone through these experiences.

However, the problem with the way young people might interact with the media, including social media, is that it can sometimes produce knee-jerk reactions which can make them very vulnerable in a space which does not support them. Say for instance, if they begin to talk about what they've been through (as many young people do on social media), they might get all kinds of reactions from the larger community. And all of that is not going to be supportive and understanding. There are so many who have faced enormous backlash for what they have shared or talked about.

One of the biggest things in trauma and abuse is that young people understand intuitively, and rightly so, that if they talked about what they went through, not many people will believe them. So when somebody, say a young teenage girl says, *'This uncle of mine did this to me when I was eight'*, most people in the family will turn around and say, *'That's impossible — he's such a nice guy'*

That kind of a response to trauma and abuse is rampant, across the board, across society, across the world. There is this feeling that they will not be believed. Or

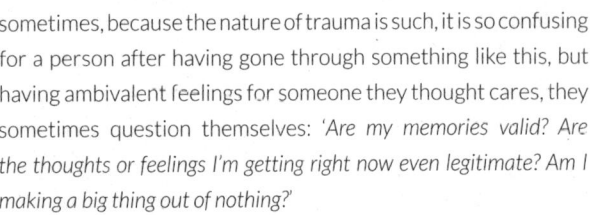

Young
MENTAL HEALTH

sometimes, because the nature of trauma is such, it is so confusing for a person after having gone through something like this, but having ambivalent feelings for someone they thought cares, they sometimes question themselves: *'Are my memories valid? Are the thoughts or feelings I'm getting right now even legitimate? Am I making a big thing out of nothing?'*

Those are the kinds of things many young people go through, and that makes it very confusing. So when there are spaces in social media or other places where people suddenly get an opportunity to talk about it and remember things, and if it is a spontaneous outpouring of grief and trauma and all that, unfortunately the response to that is often not very positive or healing to the person. That's as a word of caution.

But it is very important to address it and to help young people figure it out, and give them spaces which are safe — within the family, the larger community, schools, colleges, agencies, helplines they can access. As a society we need to figure out where will these kids go when they begin to remember things which have happened to them?

AMRITA: If you were to take the onus away from the kids/survivors, what would your advice be to friends or family? What would your advice be to someone who's not an expert and one step away from say, taking them to a counsellor ... how do we listen better and provide that support when we're not trained as counsellors?

DR AMIT SEN: It's something that is happening already, there are schools and colleges which are creating such spaces which are not judgmental, which are supportive, of people who will actually listen and take things at face value. To start with, if somebody is reporting abuse, the message to the community must be, please take it at face value.

Then figuring out how it happened, when it happened, what needs to be done, can be the next sequential steps you can take. Right at the beginning you have to believe the person when they come up with something like this.

Many times memories from childhood are not very coherent, because of the nature of how memories are formed and how children look at the world. That doesn't necessarily mean the child is lying or fabricating these things. It only means they are not able to pull it all together right now. If you help them, maybe they will be able to, and even if they don't, there is truth in some of the experiences that they have had and how you interpret them needs to be thought through.

To begin with, there needs to be empathy, there needs to be acceptance of what the person is coming up with. And that is the biggest thing we need to provide or inculcate in society, in persons at various walks of life.

We have to understand and accept that this is a part of our reality — that it happens to many children, that it's not a minority, and is probably a majority. If you look at a survey done by the Government of India and published on the site of the Ministry of Women and Child Development, they concluded that more than 80 per cent suffered some form of abuse or another.[19] This was tens of thousands of kids who were surveyed across the country, in 12 states or something like that — massive data they generated. These were children from all walks of life — children

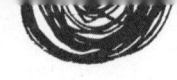

Young
MENTAL HEALTH

from middle class families, from deprived families, children living in residential homes, street kids, everything. The biggest thing was there was not a lot of difference between kids living in so-called intact, middle class families and street kids — their experience of abuse and neglect and all of that was not very different. That's shocking, isn't it? We believe we're keeping our kids safe and those are realities we have to come to terms with. As a society, in a family, as a school you'll often read or see that if there is a disclosure of abuse, particularly sexual abuse, immediately people get polarised. Schools protect their teachers and say this can't happen in our school. They will not talk to the media, they will ostracise or denounce the family, and blame the family and say it must have happened at home, and so on.

This splitting that happens is very common. Because if as a society, as a people, we have to accept that we can't protect our children, it's a very jarring realisation isn't it? It makes you feel very small and inadequate, isn't it? And that's why it's so hard to accept.

There is a phenomenon called gaze aversion, where you don't look at things which are really jarring and traumatic and painful, you turn your head away. It happens when you look at an accident in the street, you don't want to look at it, you turn your head away. With street children at your window, most people will look into their phones, they don't have the courage to look into their eyes. And I think partly it's because we know it's our responsibility – what are we doing for these kids? Those are all instances of gaze

aversion, and it happens when children come out with disclosure ... or memories of trauma, it becomes very jarring for people and very painful for them to accept.

AMRITA: For these older age groups, you've mentioned social ostracisation can lead to several issues, like eating disorders, self-harm.

DR AMIT SEN: Self-harm is another big thing we see, cutting behaviours for example, and that can happen in depression, eating disorders, trauma, and also self-harm of a larger degree, actual suicidal thoughts, planning and attempts.

We know we are one of the countries with the highest suicide rates among young people — as mentioned in the article Dr Vikram Patel and co. wrote in *The Lancet*[20] — every hour one young person kills themselves in the country. Every hour! And these are only the ones which are recorded. There are many which are not. Again, suicide comes with so much social stigma and typically the reaction of the families and community is to cover it up, isn't it.

AMRITA: That's something you also see when people come in — obviously a huge issue and something we are societally uncomfortable talking about. But when you have someone come in, how does it usually present itself? Is it usually a parent bringing in a child or a teacher or does it come out in another session?

DR AMIT SEN: Sometimes we have an urgent referral because a young person has made a suicide attempt or is clearly expressing suicidal ideas which alarms people when it comes up in the family.

In the majority (of cases), we have children who may be suffering from depression or anxiety, trauma or so on, and during therapy, when they begin to trust therapists,

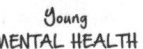

they begin to open up and talk about it, and then they start talking about how they're actually cutting themselves in places which aren't easily seen and ... having serious suicidal thoughts. They'll also add that, *'You can't share this with my parents, they'll stop me going out or they'll be devastated'*, and various other reasons. As a clinician it becomes a tricky balancing act on when to break that confidentiality. When the risks are very high, we have to take the support and help from the family and many other stakeholders, and we do that often and effectively.

Schools are an important stakeholder. Sometimes schools are supportive, but some of the top schools of the city (like international schools and so on) say, 'We can't have this child (who's expressed suicidal thoughts) anymore, it's dangerous, a risk to her and other people.'

Hearteningly, there are other schools, some of the well-known schools in Delhi, which go out of the way to say, 'We will support this child,' and add, 'We will have a school counsellor, two or three teachers and a bunch of kids who might look out for the kid.' They're really supportive ... and that's necessary.

There is a period of crisis intervention, say when the risks are really high, when it's touch and go, it's possibly a few days or even a couple of weeks when the suicidal risk is very high. Perhaps it's okay to keep the child in a very safe environment at that time. But you can't begin to exclude children just because they're harming themselves.

The other thing to understand with self-harm is that many times cutting behaviour is done with different motives and objectives. There are so many kids who say, 'We are going through so much pain and anguish, when we cut, it helps me to feel better, it actually releases the tension and anger and the upset.' And, of course, that doesn't mean we take it lightly — this kind of self-harm can lead to more serious forms of self-harm. It's important to accept it and analyse what leads to it.

Just as abuse is so common, so is suicidal behaviour and self-harm. And we can't exclude these people from our everyday life. That's, let's say, one fourth or 15–20 per cent (of our students)! There was a recent survey across the world of first-year students, in an American university, and they found that 35 per cent of kids were clinically depressed.[21] Thirty five per cent!

And perhaps a significant number of those kids would have thoughts of self-harm or would be indulging in self-harm in some form or the other. So you can imagine the numbers. It's a part of life now, so you can't say that every time a child expresses something like this, rather than help and support the child you exclude them from the mainstream of school and society. We have to support them. Here's another message for the community: we can't turn our heads away from this. This is the reality and we have to deal with this now. There could be many reasons why depression has increased so much, and we could look at prevention as well, but once the process of slipping into depression and self-harm starts, you have to include these kids.

AMRITA: One of the bigger issues people also have is how do they know they should be reaching out for professional help? Who do they reach out to? A parent or a sibling or a friend at school? What do you think are some of the warning signs?

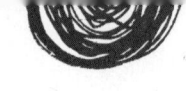

Especially for say, self-harm, since it's often done in hidden places?

DR AMIT SEN: If someone is cutting themselves or expressing suicidal thoughts, you have to reach out for professional help. But even otherwise, it should be done if there are very clear changes in the person's moods and behaviours. Now this happens often in a person's adolescent years and many times teachers and parents get confused and they will say, 'Isn't this a part of teenage?' And indeed it could be. But if the disturbances are persistent and makes a person dysfunctional in many ways, like whether it's about taking care of themselves, or regulating their own emotional life, or falling out with friends at a rapid pace, or not being able to cope with pressures in school, all those kinds of things. If they begin to happen persistently over a period of time, say over a few weeks, it's important to address it and say:

'What's happening here?'

There are many people in the community who are equipped to probably have a close look at this and figure out whether they require any further professional help from a mental health professional. That could be a school counsellor or someone in the family who has an idea or awareness of this, or a family doctor — sometimes paediatricians are very good at picking this out. It's important that this is done without feeling stigmatised and very awkward about it — it's easy to say but it's very difficult for many people to do this. Most parents and families turn around and say,

'I couldn't imagine my child going through this, she was so functional', or 'He was so good at this. How could it happen? It's never happened in my family.' That shock and dismay that something like this is happening to us or to one's own child is intense. Often people tend to deny it for some time, so they think it's a part of teenage or it will just go away and so on.

AMRITA: Since you and Dr Shelja Sen are the subject matter experts who other people come to for advice, as parents how has this impacted your parenting style?

DR AMIT SEN: We often have joked about it, when you go home as parents, all your insights and knowledge goes out the window. You're like any other parent. As parents, we have made mistakes, both Shelja and I have, and have learned from it too. Shelja's book on parenting has probably been largely from to her experiences, not just seeing children who come to us with referrals and all, but also from our own children.

It's not been a cakewalk or easy. We've had our own challenges. If you have read Shelja's first book on parenting (*All You Need is Love: The Art of Mindful Parenting*), it often talks about how parenting is about growing up ourselves as human beings. The challenges it throws at you, if you don't reflect on your own responses and what it's doing to you emotionally, then you may not be able to respond to the child's needs, particularly when it's complex and dynamic, as it is mostly. And often more so, when a child is non-neurotypical — that creates its own set of difficulties for parents.

Particularly with our older one, as we were learning on our job, so to say, we often joked and said, 'You were our guinea pig.' And he's nice enough now that he's about 20, to forgive us for it mostly … we hope. But we've made our mistakes.

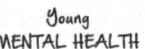
Young
MENTAL HEALTH

AMRITA: Most parents will feel it resonates. Shelja writes so openly. Even with our first book, *Real Stories of Dealing With Depression*, we've had people coming back. One parent said he didn't even realise what kind of pressure he was putting on his child. Sometimes hearing these stories helps reinforce some of the messages. Was there anything you took to heart early on, especially when your kids were younger?

DR AMIT SEN: One of the first realisations I had as a parent was that so often I bring back things from other spheres of life, let's say work, and I bring it home, and how that affects the kids. Our son, who is very perceptive, while he was no more than three or something, actually pointed that out to me. He said, 'Baba why are you feeling so grrrummph today?' And I said, 'Am I?'

And that moment I thought, 'Yes I am very troubled today,' because of something that might have happened at work. And I was trying to be nice to him on the surface, but he picked it up like that, like a sponge. And I realised that whatever you do on the surface, if your response is not actually genuine from within, kids will pick it up.

And that's one of the earliest kinds of realisations — that a lot of parenting is about genuineness, honesty, about being authentic. There are many people who have a bad marriage and they say, with very good intention, that, 'We decided not to separate because of our children', and that, 'We don't fight in front of them.'

But kids pick it up. If they're fighting behind closed doors, or if they're coming out from their room in a certain mood, that can also be traumatic for children.

That's another realisation I think I had fairly early — if you're feeling disturbed yourself, it may not be a great idea to negotiate or engage with your children. The best thing to do would be to walk away and go sort yourself out and come back.

Chapter 3
IN THEIR OWN WORDS:
LEARNING TO HEAL
By Ishita Mehra

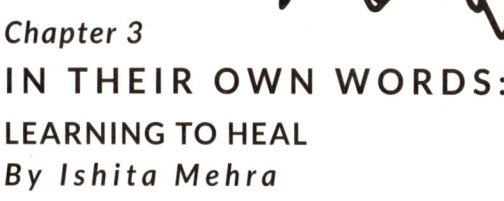

About the Artist: Ishita Mehra is a young mental health advocate and illustrator. Her work includes writing and illustrating personal stories of people about their mental health struggles, illustrating mental health themes and subjects and initiating workshops on mental health. Currently, she is focusing on starting a support group in Pune to allow people to access and facilities on mental health care. You can find her on Instagram @VoiletHill.

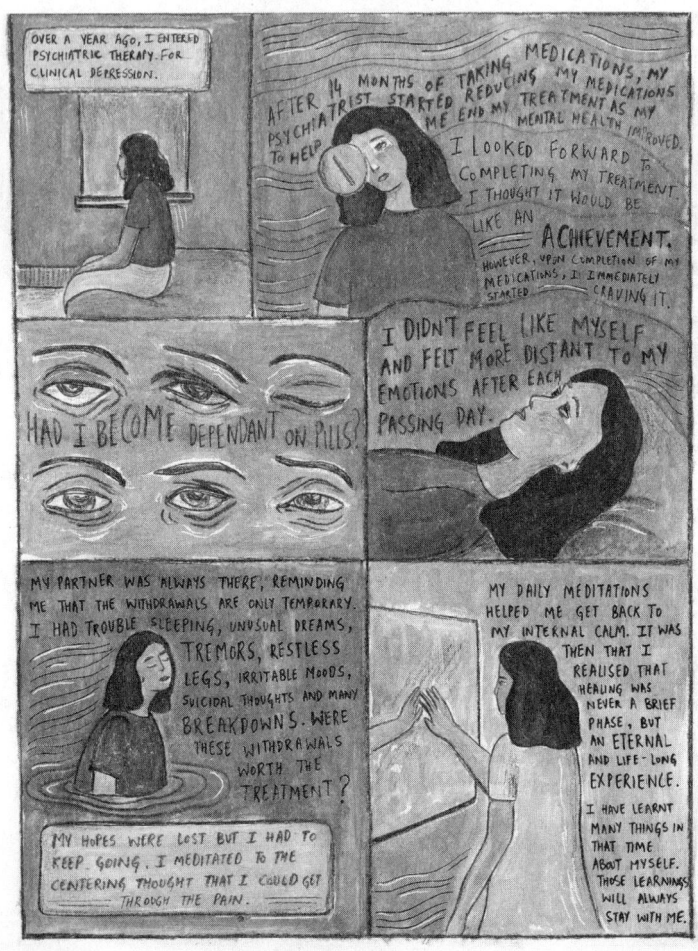

Art by Ishita Mehra for The Health Collective

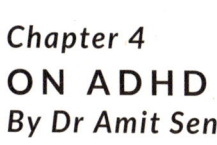

Chapter 4
ON ADHD
By Dr Amit Sen

I think one[22] of the most relevant topics today in child mental health is ADD OR ADHD (Attention Deficit Hyperactivity Disorder). It's one of the most common disorders in childhood although there is a lot of controversy still across the world about the nature of it, whether it exists at all ... about how people get over-medicated in some countries (particularly in the West). There is still an ongoing debate ... however if you see the scientific literature and wide scale studies by the WHO across the world, including centres in India, you will find that the prevalence of ADHD is as high as 5 per cent at least; whereas in some Western countries it is thought to be 10 per cent.[23]

So, what is ADHD, how does it look and what does it do to children?

Children with ADHD often are full of life, very creative sometimes with a range of talents. However, they have difficulty in focusing or attending to tasks that do not interest them. And clearly one of the main things that comes to the fore is when they begin to go to school because they cannot sit down and focus on academic work, which, often for most children as you might know, is mundane, it's boring.

These kids will not be able to complete their classwork, will not sit and do their homework, will make silly mistakes in their work. What confuses teachers and parents alike is that these kids, if they are interested in something — let's say in football or music or art — might do exceptionally well, and over there their focus and concentration does not fail them. And that is the key thing to understand that kids with ADHD will focus very well in areas of interest, but are not able to do so in whichever area or activity they are not interested in ... which again could be a wide range of things, and not just academics. For instance, if a child is passionate about football and you make them sit down and make a painting they will probably never finish it even when the day is over.

So, kids with ADHD have difficulties with attention which manifests in various ways, like I said — difficulty in completing tasks, getting distracted easily and as they grow up, not being able to manage their time very well, procrastinating, delaying their projects and assignments when they go to high school and so on. They are often very disorganised, they can lose things, misplace their belongings and so on.

So if you find a child or your child who is otherwise very bright and capable but is struggling with certain jobs — do not jump to labelling them as being lazy or careless, or *he just doesn't care and he doesn't want to do these things*, because children usually will do things they can! And if they are not able to do something, or if they are not doing something, although they might find reasons for it, it could be that they are incapable, at least at that juncture, to do it. It's important to understand this aspect from a point of view of development or neuro-development.

The other features of ADD and ADHD are hyper-activity and impulsive behaviour. So, a child who is young may have difficulty sitting still, may be very jumpy and restless and fidgety... may talk excessively, may be very loud and noisy in play areas or even at home, or sometimes at school even. They might have difficulty waiting for their turn, they might be easily frustrated, get bored very easily and so on.

And when you see some of these features in children do question whether they are wired differently to the extent that they might have something that interferes with their overall growth and development.

So, of course, you might argue that many children are like that and many children are jumpy, fidgety — but that's because they are children! However, children with ADHD after a certain time, begin to find the common developmental goals — let's say, like academics or peer relationships or self-regulation — difficult to do. When these things become dysfunctional and we find that a child that otherwise seems intelligent and capable is unable to do these things, we then suspect ADHD.

There is a wide range of therapies that are available for it — medication being one of them. Also be aware as parents, as teachers, that when you suspect a child has ADHD or send them for evaluation for ADHD, it is not mandatory to put them on medication. Because a lot of times parents particularly and sometimes teachers or schools fear this and therefore they are often very hesitant to go down that route, the medical route or the psychological route. And that's the other thing that we must remember — there is a solution.

The kind of children that we get in our centre at Children First — and we get hundreds of children with ADHD — are often very bright kids. But rather than

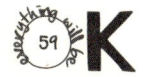

seeing their strengths and their intelligence, people have begun to criticise them or have been criticising them over a period of years, seeing only their negative traits, so they turn up in front of us with very negative stories and negative narratives of their lives and that, we believe, is more damaging than the ADHD itself. These kids then begin to get into depression and anxiety, some of them start taking substances to relieve some of this distress and some others may rebel hugely, and then be termed as having a conduct disorder or be anti-social and so on and so forth.

There's no question that if we do not treat ADHD well it can become extremely complicated and indeed become dangerous because kids who are not treated well by the school, the education system, by parents or their peers often take the other route and then they begin to identity with groups of other kids who may be doing things which are anti-social.

There is evidence again to show that if we do treat children early with ADHD, that often has a very positive outcome. Our experience of treating ADHD has been wonderful and we have so many children who are doing exceptionally well with their lives, going to the best universities, pursuing off-beat careers of maybe being divers, or mountain climbers, or musicians, or actors and doing so well. It's a great journey that you witness when you begin to see these kids from a different lens and see how capable they are rather than what they cannot do.

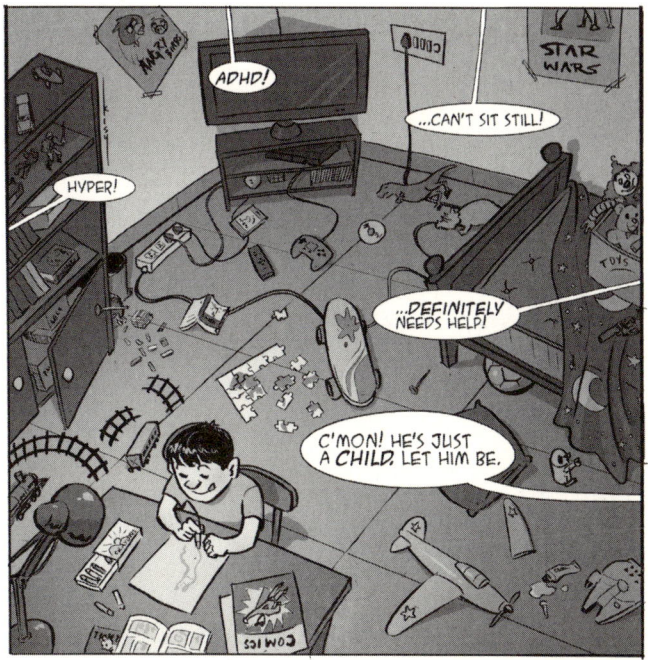

AMRITA TRIPATHI, KISHORE MOHAN | HEALTH COLLECTIVE

Artist: Kishore Mohan

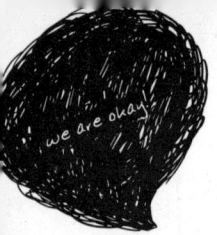

IN THEIR OWN WORDS
By Dr Sen

The Children First website says that Dr Amit Sen 'proudly believes that he has ADHD'. I asked him to share a bit more of his own journey.

On a more personal note...

I feel blessed with people around me who not only care deeply, but also look out for me whenever I stumble. They even take pre-emptive steps to prevent me from getting into trouble, both at home and at work. Shelja (my wife Dr Shelja Sen) pays all my bills before they are too late, and reminds me to pay salaries (which is my job at home and work); she helps me to complete PPTs at the eleventh hour, reminds me to put all the essentials in my bag when I'm travelling alone, and sends me numerous references and her own writings when I've crossed the deadline for an article that I'm writing.

Despite her occasional frustration, Shelja is always there and makes my functional existence sustainable. My children have learnt to live with it; my son, Nishat, has learnt to be forgiving beyond his years about my lapses, and my daughter, Anya, will respond with a roll of her eyes and an indulgent smile when I zone out during conversations.

At work, my colleague Pooja will make sure that I don't double book my appointments and exhaust myself, while Jonaki will take care to block out time in my schedule for a meeting that we have agreed on together, and Ankita will reassure me with compassion after I've forgotten to make an important call. And almost all of the rest of our wonderful team at Children First understand my limitations and are ready to scaffold me whenever I need it.

My early childhood was no different. I was the first-born on my mother's side of the family and the whole extended family couldn't have enough of this mischievous bundle of energy. They, particularly my mother, have numerous stories to tell about how she would have to try innovative methods to contain my risk-taking behaviours at 2 years of age.

For instance, tying me to the pallu (the loose end) of her saree, lest I climb the wobbly book rack or escape through the front door. Once out of the door, I would deliberately roll down the steps in order to cut time, with my mother, her saree pulled up to her knees, in hot pursuit. Such escapades would lead to frequent incidences of scraped knees and bleeding elbows, the pain of which would not deter me one bit, I am told. All these stories were recounted with a mixture of exasperation, amusement and fondness.

But things started changing in school; from as early as class 2, I remember a sinking feeling whenever a teacher would ask questions in class as I often hadn't a clue about what was being discussed. By middle school, I was increasingly struggling to complete classwork and had frequent remarks of 'Homework not done ...' by teachers in my school diary. My mother's disappointment and indignation kept growing with it and her methods of disciplining me kept getting harsher. And so did my resistance, passive aggressive at first and progressively rude and defiant as time went by.

I was quiet as a mouse in class, dodging the teachers glare, often lost in my world of fantasy and turmoil. I had started stammering when forced to speak up and my very own friends would tease and chide me in those moments. Life was tough, but what kept me going was a deep belief, despite the failure and humiliation, that I would make it one day. I have often wondered where it came from – perhaps from the early years of absolute love and nurturance, but much more from the unflinching faith that my father had in me and my abilities. Clearly not in academics, but in every other activity of interest, including football, theatre, music, food, travel and adventure, or any other novel experience that excited me. He had this naïve curiosity about whatever we (me, my brother and sister) did or brought to him, and would rejoice at every little success or discovery.

So I stumbled along through school, with my younger siblings in tow, who were equally inept at academics (it runs in the family as they say!), and was I glad to have their company. One of the dreaded times of the year was the end of March when the school final results would come out, and all the rest of our friends in the colony were, somehow, always topping their classes. On one such fateful evening, when our mother was ruing her misfortune about having such children, our father wryly quipped, "but somebody has to bring up the rear..." much to our stifled delight. Such light-heartedness and wit, and indeed playfulness, of which my mother too had dollops of, helped us all through those challenging years.

By the time I was in high school, I was gravitating towards 'bad company', though, and getting daggers from the parents of so called 'good' friends, some of whom were being asked to keep a safe distance from me. My rebellion had reached another level by then and the risk taking behaviours were indeed risky; they would make me shudder many years later, as a young parent myself, when I would remember those days. At school, the demands on my time management and organisational abilities were way beyond my bandwidth, as I could hardly ever complete my assignments on time and was scraping through the exams to somehow stay afloat from one class

to another. My frisky mind and motivation was mostly busy finding innovative ways to avoid being noticed by the teachers and prevent any contact between them and my oblivious parents, at least till the time the exam results came out. I remember clearly, with mixed feelings, the time just before school-leaving Board exams, our maths teacher demanding that I drop maths, lest I failed in it and brought the school a bad name. I stood my ground and kept shaking my head, much to her chagrin; she couldn't believe it when I eventually got a distinction in the subject. Over the years, despite the mounting pressures and gut-wrenching anxiety, I had learnt the art of scrambling to the end in the last lap of a long race (not that I recommend this strategy to anyone).

A similar approach got me into medical college. It was providence that I got into Armed Forces Medical College, an institute that was one of its kind. It had doggedly built and preserved a culture, quite in contrast to medical colleges of that era, which celebrated diversity and unconventionality. It was a community that nurtured creativity and out-of-the-box thinking, where sports, art, music and other eccentric pursuits thrived. I couldn't have found a more conducive place where football (or any sport for that matter), theatre and student politics were no longer distractions from my studies but virtues in which I could immerse myself. It was a time of rejoicing, growing up and healing. Not that the academic struggles had diminished by any means, and I continued to receive rebuke and criticism for my tardiness, poor attendance and abysmal performance in internal assessments. But somehow — perhaps through a combination of luck, pluck and ample help from wonderful friends — I managed to clear the main/professional exams in regular time.

It's truly paradoxical that I went on to get three more professional qualifications after my MBBS, each one requiring years of toil and academic performances at

regular intervals.

What kept me going, despite the frustrating procrastination and chronic belatedness, was my fascination and passion for the subject of psychiatry, and even more for child psychiatry and different forms of therapy. It opened up a world that was full of mystery, wonder and discovery.

It was during this period that it dawned on me that the struggles that I had had, through school and college, were real and not dissimilar to so many of the kids I was seeing and diagnosing with ADHD. I was not stupid, lazy or callous as I had often been called or labelled in the past, but found it genuinely challenging to be consistent and to do certain tasks that were expected of me. Such experiences of being chastised, excluded and pigeon-holed are ever so common for most kids and adults with ADHD, often leaving profound imprints in their psyche and their sense of self, or the lack of it.

I can safely admit now that it has taken me years of introspection and healing to overcome the deep sense of inadequacy and self-doubt that I carried for decades.

Shelja would say, half in jest, that for a person with ADHD to have a fulfilling life, they need a profession that they love and a life partner that gets them. Fortunately, I have both.

As we always say, to parents and teachers, at the end of each ADHD workshop – 'keep the faith...'

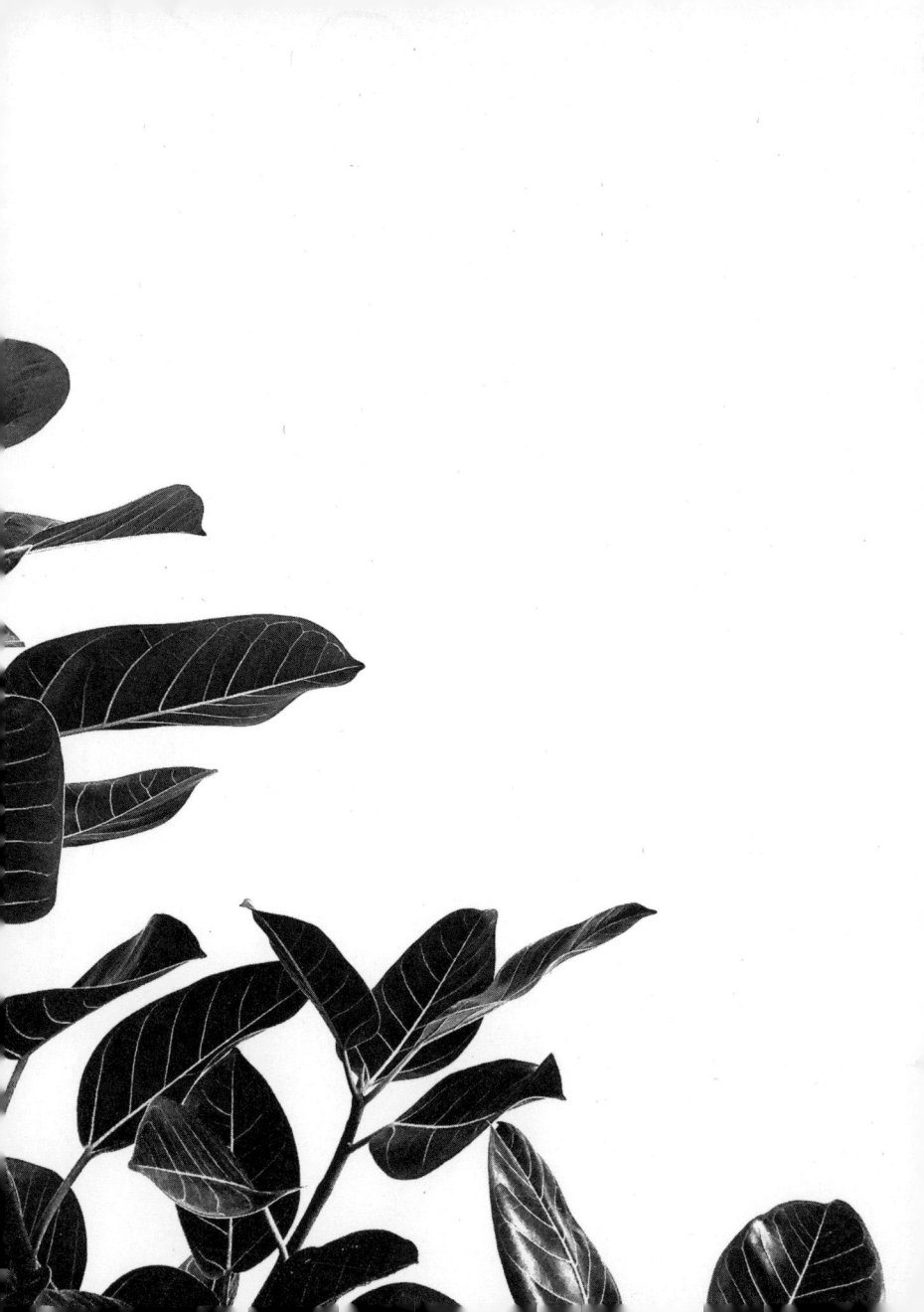

Chapter 5
SHARING THE STRUGGLE

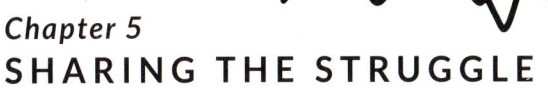

Paras Sharma is the head of The Alternative Story, a Bengaluru and Mumbai-based service that offers counselling for individuals and organisations, as well as group therapy, online therapy and an innovative 'Pay What You Want' model.

The 32-year-old grew up in what was then called Bombay, in a small suburb called Dahisar, that he describes as being in a middle/lower middle class neighbourhood. He studied at Wilson College and then at the Tata Institute of Social Sciences (TISS). Paras has been in practice for approximately a decade, and was earlier programme coordinator at the TISS-housed psycho-social helpline, iCall, in Mumbai. He tweets as @wisedonkay and often shares personal accounts of his own struggles, including with anxiety. Here are lightly edited excerpts of an interview.

Young MENTAL HEALTH

AMRITA: Drawing on your professional experience at The Alternative Story and previously at iCall, what do you think are the primary mental health/illness concerns for young Indians?

PARAS SHARMA: My perspective on the mental health concerns that young Indians are facing has shifted quite a bit since I graduated about 10 years ago. About 10 years ago, I would probably just parrot the same statistics that were mentioned in our text books — it's probably depression, anxiety, etc. I don't think about it like that anymore, simply because I have worked in two spaces which are primarily community mental health ... and I think my teaching experience also has changed my perspective quite a bit. I think there's an important point here that we need to make — that there is definitely a distinction between mental health concerns people are facing and mental illness concerns people are facing, especially young people.

I say this because my praxis is now anchored primarily in a post-modern, intersectional feminist and existential lens, where the emphasis is laid on the context being a toxic one, rather than the individual being pathological. When we say the context is toxic or pathological, we are taking away responsibility from the individual. So definitely there is fatigue, burn-out, isolation... worry, anxiety, lack of meaning, lack of fulfilment, which are all experiences which are nearly universal for young people right now. And all of this can — and sometimes does not also — lead to mental illness.

But I think that the fact that we feel low, lonely, worthless, hopeless, anxious, unable to relax and generally very pessimistic and cynical about our futures is a normative experience. In Existential Psychotherapy, we call this Normative Anxiety because we are saying that life is the stressor, we are not saying that there is a need for other stressors, just the challenges of life, especially in a transitional generation. When we say transitional generation, it usually is the generation which is sandwiched between growing up with one set of norms and facing a different set of norms when they have grown up.

So the millennial generation especially is one where it is like this — we know both the pre-technology and technology era together. A lot of the norms which we were told we should imbibe and follow when we were children don't hold true anymore for us. A lot of the concerns that we have today are because of institutions that we took for granted, and our parents took for granted not being there for us anymore. So the path that we were told we should be taking as individuals is simply not there anymore. Primarily, I think these are the concerns young people are facing. This is as much a mental health concern as it is a political concern. Because you know, what's going to happen to a millennial today when they get out of college? What are the jobs awaiting us? What are the residential spaces available to somebody? What is the kind of lifestyle and healthcare that a person is going to be able to access?

If you take a look at people who are not in the Tier 1 cities, not studying at the Tier 1 institutions, if you look at people in smaller towns, studying at Tier 3, Tier 4 colleges, the job prospects for them are extremely poor. The mental health concerns I think are innately tied to the fact that this is what is happening in the context around us. And I definitely believe that any mental illness that comes out of this is solely because of the context, and not because of the individual. Because overwhelmingly, we are seeing that there is a disadvantage that millennials and post-millennials are going to face.

AMRITA: What are some the colloquial terms/ways people present or talk about mental health issues — whether it's stress/*tanav*/*pareshaan*/sadness/depression?

PARAS SHARMA: I think you've hit the nail on the head when you've said 'stress', 'tension' in terms of colloquial terms ... I think depression, stress, anxiety, worry and local variations of this are things that people are able to now verbalise. Depression, panic, panic attack, breakdown, are all words that have entered into the urban dwelling people's lexicon, even if it's in a vernacular language. So, I definitely think these are colloquial ways and terms with which people are expressing their mental health concerns.

I think one more thing that we need to look at is there are physical health concerns which are often presented ... and these are primarily mental health concerns which are misrepresented as physical health concerns. Just to give you some context on my own experience for that matter. For me it started off — my mental health journey of getting a diagnosis and starting medication — with strong feelings of fatigue, poor sleep and an inability to fall asleep even after being very tired and having done a full day's work. So people are coming to us with physical health presentations, and those are the terms that people are finding accessible and talking about.

AMRITA: What kick-started your interest in mental health? And can you share a bit of your personal journey?

PARAS SHARMA: I think it's a process that slightly dates back to the time that I was finishing school. I knew that I wanted a career in humanities when I got out of school so that was very, very clear. I wasn't happy with the lack of emphasis that people would pay to social sciences and languages — those were my favourite subjects in school. Everybody was oriented towards math and science, and I generally did not like that. I was very clear I would get into humanities. When I got into humanities, I was suddenly given an option to study entirely new subjects which I was never offered in school — psychology, philosophy, French — subjects which were not ever given as options to me in a state board school. When I started learning psychology in Class XI, I knew that was something that I really, really enjoyed. I think now I realise a lot of my early anxiety-like symptoms were around maths and science exams, which I didn't really enjoy at all. When I started studying these subjects — literature, philosophy, psychology — it was like a weight had been lifted and I enjoyed my studies and I think those years in college were really the best ones for me.

I think literature, philosophy and psychology, which were my subjects in my undergrad, were a really good, well-put together combination, because psychology borrows a lot from philosophy, literature borrows a lot from philosophy, so there is a lot of interplay, of references between all of these three subjects.

I feel the journey for being a counselling psychologist began when our college introduced a counselling psychologist on campus, and I started seeing people going to the counsellor, talking about going for counselling, and saw that people were actually helped. At that time, there was a psychology department and a society which was started and I attended the talk and came to know what counselling was, and I really thought that this is something that I want to look at as I go ahead.

By the time I came to the final year, I was pretty sure I wanted to pursue psychology and I wanted to continue either in the field of counselling psychology or social psychology, because primarily, I wanted to work with people in terms of behavioural and emotional well-being. At that point, the discourse of community mental health was not something that I was familiar with. But I think coming to a place like TISS for my studies was a great fortune for me, because it very neatly tied the social work discourse with the mental health discourse for me. For me, the two are inseparable. I can't see mental health as separate from community work. So I think that's how it has started for me.

I did my Master's in 2009–11 and I started working in hospitals as a medical social worker, raising funds, and counselling people pre, post and during their surgery (not the people, but their families). That's what I was basically doing in the first couple of years, and then I was invited by my department at TISS to come and interview for this post of programme coordinator for iCall, which I was really happy to do because I was looking at doing something involving core mental health at that point in time, and it worked out and I think it was one of the best things that ever happened to me. I spent a good, happy four and a half years over there and then I moved to Bangalore, knowing fully well that I wanted to start something of my own. And it took me about a year to figure that out and finally take the leap to start The Alternative Story, so that's where I am now in the work I'm doing.

AMRITA: You have said in the past that being open about some of your struggles has helped clients/folks connect with you. Can you share a bit more?

PARAS SHARMA: I think when I started off with The Alternative Story, I was definitely going for counselling as an individual, but I was not living with mental illness or diagnosed mental illness at that time. Of course I had mental health challenges. When I started talking about my own struggles as a therapist, you know, in terms of trying to do something independent in a predominantly start-up city, wherein I don't fit into the for-profit-ness of the start-up culture and I don't fit into the non-profit, privileged circles which are very, very small, very, very incestuous. That was a very isolating experience. I started having these anxieties, these concerns, these health breakdowns, and eventually these mental health breakdowns, I decided to talk about them, I didn't want to hold back. I continued talking about my struggles, my challenges on social media and eventually I spoke about how I took time off and went on medication. That's been something that has primarily helped people connect with me.

I still use it as a tool to connect with clients, students, friends, acquaintances, because it's refreshing to see someone that's not just telling you, You should go on meds, 'but is able to tell you as a person, I'm on meds', that this is the real picture ... that it's not all magical, but it's not all doom and gloom like you hear in these horror stories about meds. I think that's helped me in connecting with people.

AMRITA: What was the driving force behind setting up The Alternative Story and can you share more about the 'Pay What You Want' model?

Young
MENTAL HEALTH

PARAS SHARMA: When I worked for funded NGOs in the past, backed by influential funders and supported by big corporates, we still saw that there were difficulties in meeting the demand of services that was out there. When I came to Bangalore, I was working for an out-and-out cut-throat for-profit, and I did not relate to that. I felt that there is a necessity for something in the middle, because the NGO sector is saturated and burnt out, and at the for-profit, people were just bored and frustrated because we were not getting enough work, although there were so many people in the organisation.

So I saw this lop-sidedness — that people who are providing services for free are few and over-loaded, and people who are providing services on a paid basis are many and very, very expensive. So I knew something low-cost, but not free, would mean that a larger number of people would be able to access the service. The idea of taking from the privileged and subsidising for the under-privileged is an essential part of the community mental health discourse.

So 'Pay What You Want' evolved out of this idea that there is no one price for people to afford therapy — different people have different prices at which they can afford therapy. So I said, let's just keep it as low as possible as an entry point and let's do the math, of how many individuals can I support in order to make a certain amount that I want, to give myself a living wage. So I decided I'll keep it at ₹199 because that was a price point which made sense for me and was not very different from what NGOs and places like NIMHANS were charging at that point in time. So I said Rs 199 would be the entry or base rate that we would look at, and my workings were such that I could do 25 per cent of my time doing sessions at Rs 199 and the rest at full price in order to be able to break even and pay myself a living wage.

And I said, let's take a chance on this and do it, and what I realised was that there were a lot of takers for it, and surprisingly, people were not paying Rs 199!

People were paying more than that. And I didn't want to turn away somebody who wanted to pay more than that, because you know, it gives them a sense of control over what they are paying. But at the same time when people have not had money, they have been able to stretch 1,000 rupees for a month or even two months of therapy, which is fantastic, because you don't even get a full session of therapy for 1,000 rupees anymore.

So the 'Pay What You Want' model was to see how much can I do at a very low cost, even if I'm not making any money, or even losing money off of it, the larger volume of work is supposed to offset the cost of that. That's the model that we have followed and at scale, that model works really well. Because when it's three of us practising full-time, the number of people who could benefit just goes up more and more. When it was a team of four, we had between us, one full-time employee's worth of time at 'Pay What you Want' (rates), and we are not an NGO but we were still able to do this. The more the organisation grows, the more such hours become available and that's the direction in which I wanted to take the work we were doing.

That's been our journey for the last 18 months and now we have started taking on academy trainees, basically students enrolled in master's degree or post-graduate diploma programmes, who have a required component of 100+

hours during each semester. If there are students who need mentorship and training on one hand, and on the other hand, there are people who need therapy at no cost or low cost, this is the best opportunity available. So we have now started offering that, which opens up even more avenues for people to access supervised and trained therapists, while being able to afford or even access therapy for free, without making it an unsustainable venture, which is what Alt Story is doing.

AMRITA: Can you shed more light on the journey to getting help in India. People do often ask: 'Who do I turn to for help?'

PARAS SHARMA: The journey of getting help in India is a difficult one, because people first of all don't turn to the mental health professionals — because one, we don't know that there are mental health professionals. If we know there are mental health professionals, we don't know what exactly they do. And in cases where we know what they exactly do, there is a huge stigma against going there, for the very reason that we know what they do. People try families, spirituality, alternative healing, self-help, eventually physical help via alternative medicine or alternative healings and therapies and then I think, when all else fails, people say okay, this is really not helping me, what do I do. This is often the case … this is often the number of hoops people have to jump through before they come to therapy. I think that is what happens.

There are also a lot of unethical and misrepresenting

professionals out there, so that makes the process even more complicated.

I think one of the biggest things that I used to do on my Twitter page (@wisedonkay), and one of the things that has led me to take a break from it, is this incessant stream of requests for: Here are my concerns, what do I do? Here is where I am, who is a good therapist? Here is where I am, who is a good doctor? This is my friend who is in an emergency, how do I help them? I have a family member who refuses to seek any help, how do I help them?

And it's just the same questions, over and over and over again. There are no answers for these mostly because there are no services available in so many places and people have rigid mindsets quite often about what kind of help they are willing to seek, what kind of modalities they are willing to use to accept therapy. It's a difficult one to crack so I hope you can make some sense of that.

AMRITA: Who did you turn to for help?

PARAS SHARMA: I went to a therapist and when things looked like I needed medication, I went to a psychiatrist that I have closely worked with. So for me, the journey was pretty simple, because I knew and I really believed that therapy works and I also do believe that medication works when you need it. So I don't really identify with this entire thing that, 'Oh, we should always be anti-medicine'.

Medicines are needed when people need them, and they work for people who need them, so I really don't endorse a view that says you shouldn't ever go on medicines and I also don't endorse a view that medication should be the first thing that you go to.

So simply put, I went to therapy and I continue to go for therapy, and when I realised it was time for me to go on medication, I went on medication. I still think it is time for me to stay on medication, so I continue. The time when my therapist, my doctor and I feel that I'm ready to go off of it, we will start tapering it, and we will see how that goes.

AMRITA: What are myths you want to bust or a wider message you would like to spread further?

PARAS SHARMA: The last bit — that it's not the case that medication is always bad and it's not that medication is always the answer. There's a lot of grey area in between and we should respect people's opinions, choices. But I really don't believe in those who actively dissuade people from seeking therapy or seeking medication. I wholly respect my client's agency to use faith, use alternative medication, or use alternative healing practices, as long as they also continue seeking therapy and seeking medication if they need it. But I don't appreciate mental health professionals or medical professionals for not doing that, and I also don't appreciate alternative healers or spiritual practitioners or leaders who dissuade people from seeking counselling or seeking medication, calling these Western concepts. That's the myth I would really like to talk about over here.

AMRITA: What would your message to your younger self be?

PARAS SHARMA: I really don't think there's a message per se, that I'd like to give to my younger self. I don't think I would have planned my life in any other way. Of course, there are difficult experiences that I've had in my past — some days I feel if they hadn't happened, life would have been simpler. But I don't think I'd be doing the work I'm doing if not for the experiences as a child or while growing up. If there is a message at all to my younger self, it's just keep working on the thing that's there in front of you next, and you'll find your way ahead. For me, it's always been a worrisome thing to not have a path charted out or not know how it's going to go, like ten years ahead or twenty years ahead. If I can give a message to my younger self and my present self it'd also be: just work on what's there in front of you right now, and it just unfolds for you as you keep going. That's what I would like to share.

Chapter 6
ON BULLYING

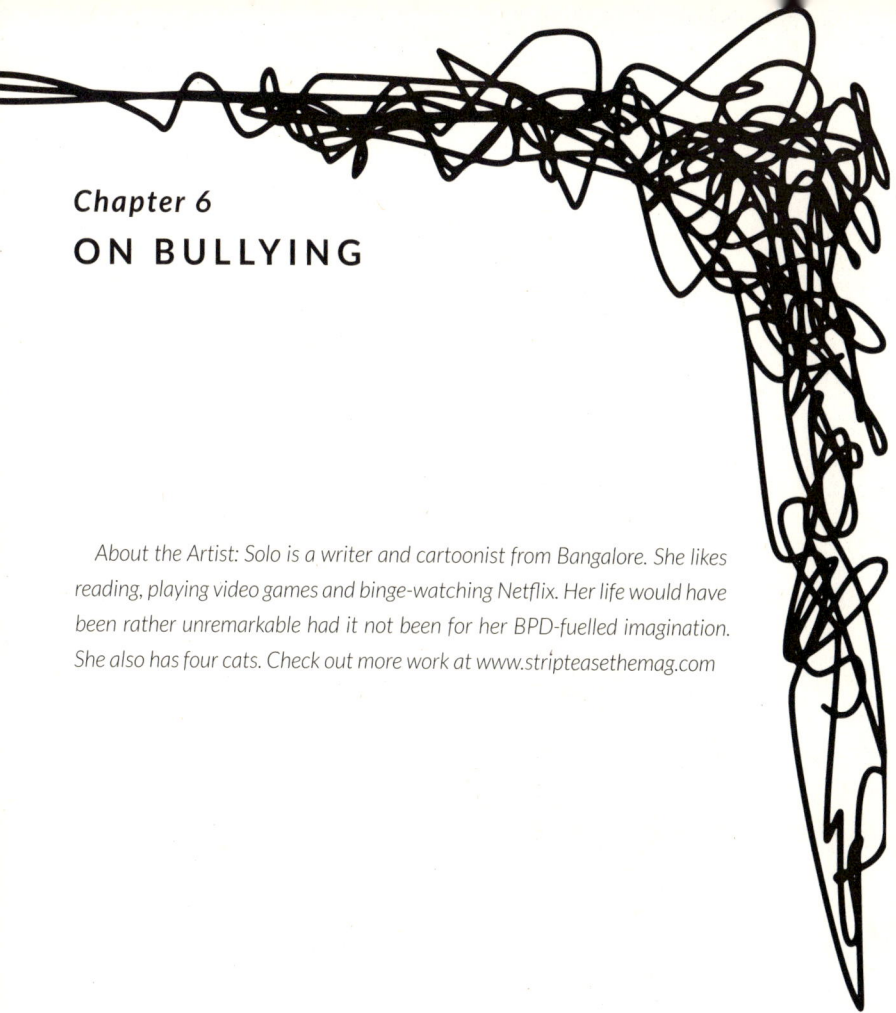

About the Artist: Solo is a writer and cartoonist from Bangalore. She likes reading, playing video games and binge-watching Netflix. Her life would have been rather unremarkable had it not been for her BPD-fuelled imagination. She also has four cats. Check out more work at www.stripteasethemag.com

Young
MENTAL HEALTH

THINGS I WISHED THEY TAUGHT YOU AT SCHOOL...

BY SOLO

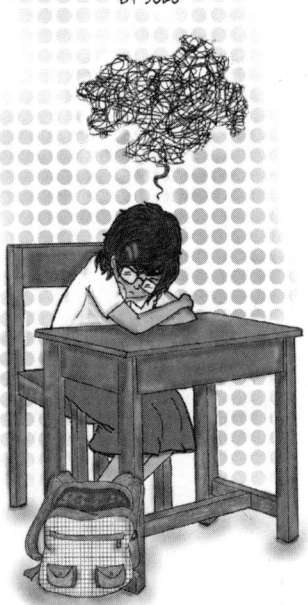

Every school has a bunch of bullies
Insufferable, and relentless.

Some make you feel bad
Because you don't ace classes

And some,
Because you can't play a sport.

Some laugh because
Your family's dysfunctional.

And some,
Because your family's poor.

Some hate you
For being fat, thin,
Even for the food you bring.

But when things feel so bad,
That you never want
To leave your room,

Never forget,
The sun hides behind the gloom.

Even though you want
To be liked,
Always remember,
No bully –
Smarter, or prettier, or richer –
Will ever be better than you.

Art by Solo for The Health Collective

BULLYING AND SCHOOL KIDS[24]
By Dr Amit Sen

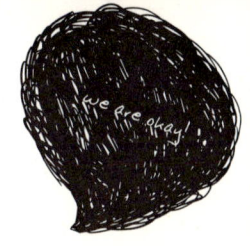

I feel bullying is hugely underestimated and a lot of people don't quite understand what it means.

Schools that say they don't have bullying — and many schools say they don't have any bullying in their campuses — probably don't understand what it entails. Bullying is rampant across cultures, across different age groups and socio-cultural spaces, so it's not just in schools, though in schools it's most common and is one of the central things that affects mental health in children.

Bullying can be categorised into three broad categories:

- **Physical Bullying**: Most apparent, people can recognise this because it's out there
- **Emotional Bullying**: This often goes unnoticed because of the nature of it
- **Cyber-bullying**: This is increasingly becoming damaging to young people

The emotional part is hard to catch on to, there is an undercurrent to such bullying that happens right from the time children are in junior school. This happens in the form of name-calling, teasing, ostracising someone, starting a rumour or scandal about somebody — all of that constitutes emotional bullying and that happens all the time in pretty much all our schools.

Cyber bullying is increasing beyond our comprehension and beyond our control.

The signs of bullying are varied and sometimes children who are otherwise well-settled in school might begin to refuse to go to school. They might begin to show signs of anxiety like stomach pain or vomiting in the morning, or they might get distracted in class, or start having other signs of depression, or start crying very easily. They might also begin to withdraw from playing areas, social spaces, become irritable, have mood swings, the younger ones might start bed-wetting. There are a wide range of symptoms.

Particularly for a child who is otherwise well-adjusted in school and begins to show these symptoms, one of the things we should always consider as parents, as school teachers is — is the child getting bullied? And then look into it, look into relationships, look into what an older child might have got on a mobile phone — of course with their permission!

Since bullying is so real and prevalent, there's no question that it has to be treated with seriousness and a zero tolerance approach.

KINDNESS IS COOL
Affirmation by Adwaita Das

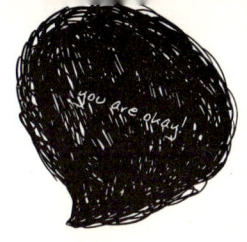

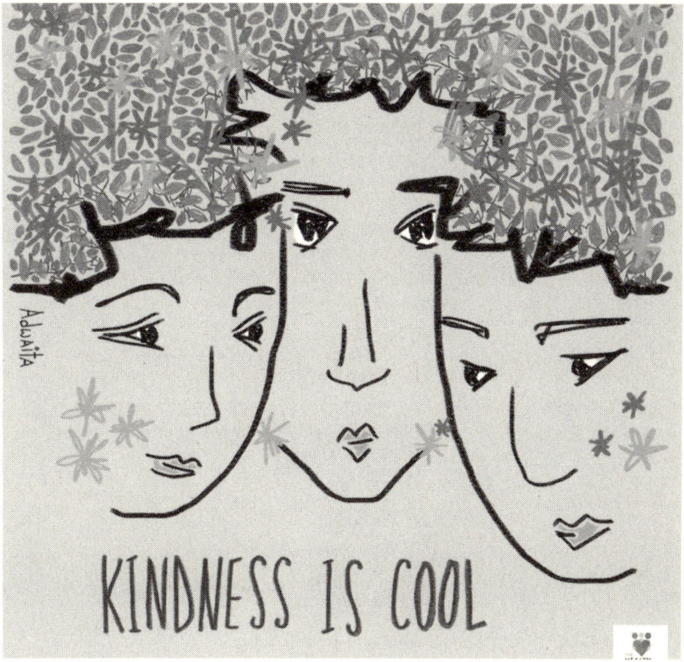

About the Artist: Adwaita Das is an author-filmmaker-artist from Planet Earth. Her book of stories - Colours of Shadow *- and books of poetry -* 27 Stitches *and* Songs of Sanity *- deal with the human psyche.* Karon Kolkata Ebong Onyo Golpo, *her anthology film, is ready for release. She creates art for mental wellness. Currently she's writing an epic sci-fi-fantasy.*

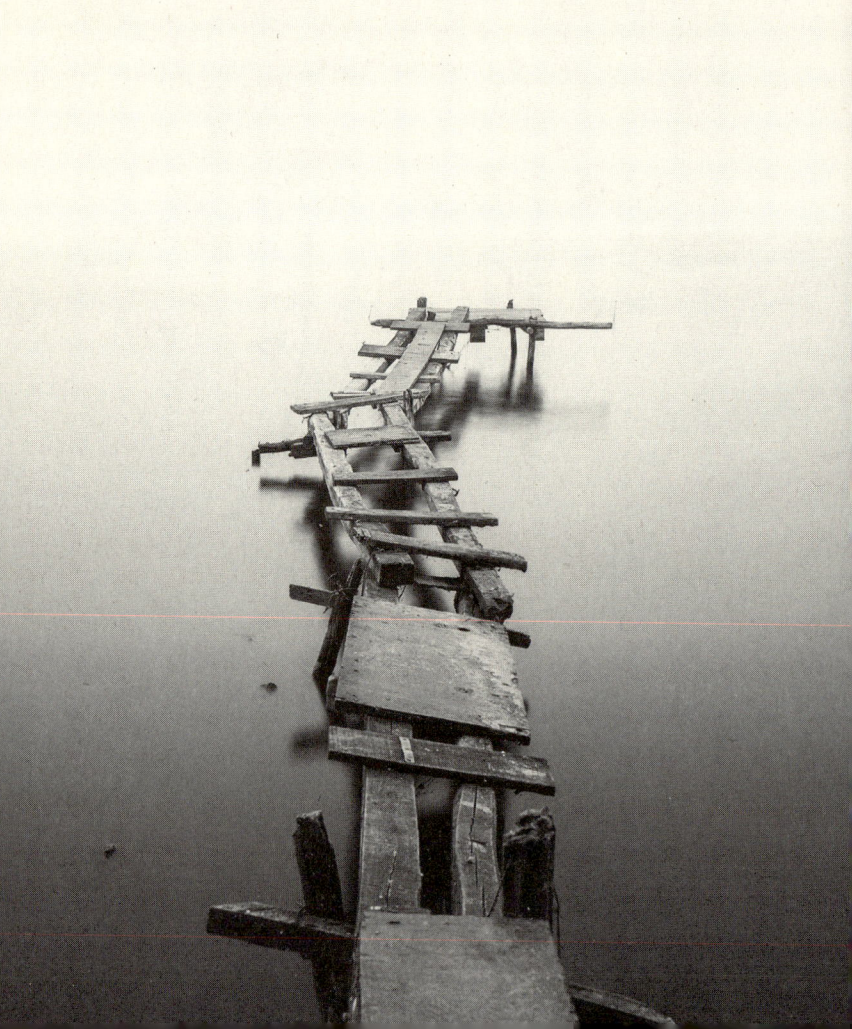

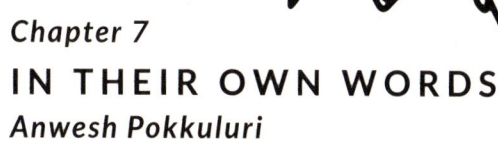

Chapter 7
IN THEIR OWN WORDS
Anwesh Pokkuluri

Anwesh Pokkuluri is the pinnacle of the Indian dream, in some ways — a young IIT graduate no less, who took on the broader legal system, leading a group of other IITians to file a petition against Section 377 in the Supreme Court. But he's had a tough path to get here — not knowing who to confide in while growing up, and always feeling a huge amount of pressure to be 'good', even 'always smiling'.

He describes himself as being raised in a semi-orthodox family. He grew up in Kakinada, a tier-2 city in coastal Andhra Pradesh, and moved to Chennai after twelfth grade to pursue his undergraduate degree at IIT Madras, graduating in 2014. After working in data analytics for a few years, he has taken a break, is staying in Kakinada, and teaches maths and social studies part-time.

Pokkuluri shared a part of his journey with The Health Collective in August 2018[25], mere weeks before the Supreme Court's landmark judgement, decriminalising the archaic and inhumane Section 377. He has very movingly expanded on his story for this book and our readers, sharing more of his journey coming out, and dealing with extraordinary loss.

BATTLING FEAR, DEPRESSION AND THE PRESSURE TO ALWAYS BE GOOD
(Trigger warning: Suicidal ideation)

JUSTICE

In May 2018, I signed up to be a petitioner in the Supreme Court against Section 377. My parents weren't comfortable with it, even though my coming out to them two and a half years before was rather smooth (for me). They had two major apprehensions.

One, how this would affect my wellbeing, considering that I'd been on a break from work for more than a year by then, owing to mental health issues. I convinced them that I was not alone, there were other petitioners with me, that we were doing it on behalf of a 350+ member support group, and if anything, this could only have a positive impact on me.

Two, this would mean coming out publicly to extended family members and neighbours, which I might not have done otherwise. I had read somewhere once: 'Queer people coming out of the closets puts the parents in the closets.' I felt that it was a legitimate concern and I wanted to talk to my therapist about how to be okay with it.

In our conversation, my therapist asked me if I feared any backlash that I, or my parents, would have to experience. I replied: 'Anyone who has seen me in real life knows that I'm a good person and wouldn't shun me. So my parents shouldn't be afraid of ostracisation.'

I admitted that it was naive, and that homophobia was a serious issue, but I stressed again saying, 'But I'm a good person. Anyone who knows me personally knows that.' And it got me thinking why I stressed about being a good person, whether I myself still had internalised homophobia that made me think being gay was a bad thing, and if I thought being good otherwise could/should compensate for it.

When my therapist asked if there were any incidents in the past which made me feel similarly, I told him how coming out to friends sometimes reinforced this belief when they said, 'But you are cool. Things will be cool between us.'

With that talk, I realised how I'd always felt the need to be extra cautious to be good, to be smiling always, to not rub anyone the wrong way. How it was tiring to do that all the time. I told my therapist about the Alan Turing pardon in 2013 (which happened a few days after the Supreme Court of India reinstated Section 377). Turing was punished because he was gay. But he received a posthumous pardon because he was an exceptional genius. This, 46 years after homosexuality was decriminalised in England, essentially sent out the message: 'Be exceptionally good if you're gay.'

This is just one of the ways in which being gay has put a strain on my mind and mental health. Growing up in a small town with no access to any resources to understand homosexuality meant questioning everything about myself — my thoughts, my feelings — starting from when I was 11 through all of my teenage years. As a result, I could never form a sense of self — not knowing who I was, not knowing if I had a problem, not knowing what I could do, not knowing whom to talk

to or what to talk about — not knowing if I could even talk.

...

ACCEPTANCE

I grew up in Kakinada where I studied till my twelfth grade. I had noticed that I was attracted to guys when I was 11 years old and didn't know what that meant at that time. No one around talked about the changes during puberty and any kind of sexual attraction, let alone same-sex. Only mention was in conversations with the other guys which honestly never amounted to any kind of knowledge. The kind of family I grew up in, talking about attractions was strictly prohibited, and that too at an age when one had to give all they had in themselves to academics. No one ever wondered if I was odd, or becoming more silent as long as I maintained my grades. I didn't have any resources to even learn the word 'homosexuality' until I moved to IIT Madras. Hailing from a lower middle class family which couldn't afford internet, the extent of truth for me was what I saw at home and school.

Things didn't magically turn around for me even after moving to Chennai. I started learning about homosexuality — thanks to the internet — and slowly came to terms with myself, but there wasn't a conducive environment to talk about it with anyone. I never thought I would get to talk about it with anyone in the four years, but a junior of mine came out to me in my seventh semester (September 2013) which made me come out to him in reciprocation. I remember how that went though — neither of us even uttered the word 'gay', we'd both told each other we were not straight. And that was not because of a lack of understanding of the word, but the stigma associated with it. However, it was still relieving and I came out to three to four other friends after that, all of them received it well and supported me.

Also, since there weren't any role models while growing up, I spent all my teenage years in confusion, helplessness, anger and denial; but if there was one emotion that was central to all of it, it was fear. Fear that I might be kicked out of school, or college, or that my parents might disown me, if either of them ever got to know about it.

The first time I had gone to a psychiatrist was in my final year at college (January 2014). After maintaining a near 100 per cent attendance for the first six semesters, I found it hard to get out of bed and go to classes in my seventh semester. On the surface, it looked like I had valid reasons to be anxious or low — I was unhappy with my summer internship (May–July 2013), I was worried about the placement interviews at the end of the seventh semester (December 2013), I had to pull out of the college student body elections at the last minute (March 2013), I was anxious about a big change in life — moving from college to work. It started affecting my diet and sleep too, and how I interacted with friends — I was always low on energy and lying about why I wasn't showing up for classes or to hang out.

When I realised I wasn't nearly as relieved as I had expected to be after I got placed, I felt that the un-motivation and anxiety during the semester had more reasons than I had thought, and that it might be a good idea to go to a counsellor. I made an appointment with the psychiatrist at the campus hospital and visited her, but it wasn't of much help as she suggested that I should try to hang out with friends more and should probably play a sport. It seemed like a very generic suggestion given without even acknowledging that I had trouble doing that. I didn't visit her or any other professional again in college, and didn't even mention that to anyone.

Right after college, two weeks before my convocation and the beginning of work, my younger brother (two years younger) passed away (July 2014). It was a sudden death. He had an ischemic stroke, went into a coma and died within hours. It was devastating for me and my parents, and I couldn't think of anything else after that for months. I was worried about my parents and wondered how to protect them while trying to deal with the loss myself. By that time, I had reached the stage of self-acceptance regarding my sexuality, had come out to a few close friends, and had plans to come out to my parents, but it felt extremely selfish to put them through that after they had just lost a son. I wondered what expectations they had of me considering I was their only child. And I started beating myself up for not being able to give them what they might wanted, and wondering if I was even a good son. Caught between the inability to deal with the loss and blaming myself for what had been happening believing it would have been better if I had died instead of my brother, I started isolating myself from friends and family. I felt very undeserved. It became overwhelming after a while and I developed suicidal thoughts.

(Note: If you or someone you know is feeling suicidal or has expressed such thoughts please reach out for professional help. You can find helplines at the end of this book.)

I became dysfunctional by July 2015 and I realised I needed to seek help again. My best friend from college made an appointment with a psychiatrist and even accompanied me to the first few visits.

My parents had already noticed that I was struggling and was unable to share things with them so they felt relieved when I told them I went to a psychiatrist. They said, 'If you can't talk to us about what is happening with you, at least talk to someone else.'

After receiving professional help for depression and anxiety, after spending hours in therapy gathering courage and vocabulary to come out to my parents, I thought it was a happy ending when they accepted me.

But the lack of sense of identity and self, with the intense lows getting normalised, my mental health remained a concern. Suicidal thoughts kept coming back. I overdosed one night after quitting work and moving back home, and had to get hospitalised. Oftentimes, the right kind of medical help seemed elusive. But again, I could at least understand the problem, look for help and was able to afford it. In the process, I realised that understanding and accepting homosexuality and mental illness are privileges.

...

CONNECTION

The first time I came out to a friend (a day after I had come out to my junior in reciprocation), we were in a class together, I scribbled on a paper that I was not straight and started crying. He told me it was okay and hugged me after the class which felt very comforting. I came out to a few close friends after that, all of them received it well and offered any support I needed. I came out to my parents in November 2015 and started coming out to more of my friends and colleagues after that. A common response from my parents and some of the friends was,
'You could have told us what was going on much earlier instead of going through it alone all these years.'

I realised that it was true, that I could have shared this truth with someone much before and even if they had not known how to accept it, it would have at least given me space to talk about it instead of having to struggle to find strength to deal with it all alone.

And the first time I talked about my mental health was at work with a colleague (July 2015). I had severe suicidal ideation one day and spent an hour in the restroom with a penknife, wanting to slit my wrists. I needed to distract myself and at that point I didn't know how to lie anymore so I took a colleague out and told her what had just happened. She talked me out of it for the time being and I visited a psychiatrist after that.

In my experience, many of the times I confided in someone about my mental health, more often than not, people could relate to what I was saying and narrated their own experiences of loneliness or the feeling of hopelessness, and also expressed how lonely it feels in those times. Many of these times, people thanked me for being vulnerable around them and said it encouraged them to open up about their own struggles. How relieving it feels when you see you're not alone! It feels like when we share our story with someone, we take on some of their strength as well to fight our battles. It's not as tiring when we don't have to fight alone.

That's why if there's anything that I can advise my younger self, it is to talk. We're only as sick as our secrets, and by talking about what is bothering us, we take away its power to control us. Be it sexuality or mental health, I wish I had opened up sooner.

The following are words from a Netflix special called Nanette by an Australian stand-up comedian Hannah Gadsby (who is queer as well and talks about mental health):

'Stories hold our cure. I just needed my story heard, my story felt and understood by individuals with minds of their own. Because, like it or not, your story ... is my

story. And my story ... is your story. I just don't have the strength to take care of my story anymore. I don't want my story defined by anger. All I can ask is just please help me take care of my story. Do you know why we have the sunflowers? It's not because Vincent van Gogh suffered. It's because Vincent van Gogh had a brother who loved him. Through all the pain, he had a tether, a connection to the world. And that ... is the focus of the story we need.'

To sum up, I would advise anyone who's feeling a lack of safety (including my younger self) to look out for people who value authenticity and can handle being vulnerable, and share their stories. More often than you'd think, you're met with understanding, comfort, relief, connection, strength. Also, we can all be vulnerable about our struggles in our everyday lives which can create a safe space for everyone.

...

HEALING

Regarding my own personal journey, I've been going to my current therapist for three years now. We've identified that I have accumulated layers of trauma, my own and intergenerational — my parents' inter-caste marriage and my mother's family disowning her, me growing up gay in denial, the sudden death of my brother, unhealthy relationships. My therapist made me see how I didn't give space to myself to process the grief of my brother's death because I was worried about how my parents were handling it and that I had to be there for them. In the process, I forgot how to emote and everything became cognitive.

My therapist started with how to identify emotions and feel them in real time, we're now working on how to change thought patterns, and how to unlearn unhealthy coping mechanisms — some of them like fight, flight, fawn (people pleasing in order to deflect from letting myself feel), freeze (dissociate, again to distract from feeling). We're working on cultivating radical acceptance towards trauma.

When I first started going to therapy — and I notice this among a lot of other people as well — I wanted a quick fix to my 'negative' emotions which had started to feel overwhelming. I believed that once I stopped feeling sad or afraid or angry, everything would work out great. Thinking we, or our emotions, need fixing feeds into a loop of believing we are broken in some way. And this not only doesn't help in our healing but also sets us on a pattern of new maladaptive mechanisms. Especially for those of us young people who have not felt adequate sense of safety while growing up and picked up unhealthy patterns in our formative years, we may question comfort and love in our later relationships, and are prone to stay in abusive relationships. It's imperative we hold space for ourselves and form support systems.

GIVE YOUR HEART TO YOURSELF

Affirmation by Adwaita Das

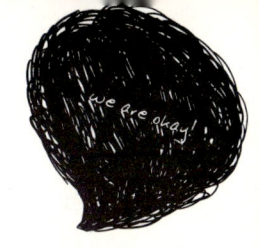

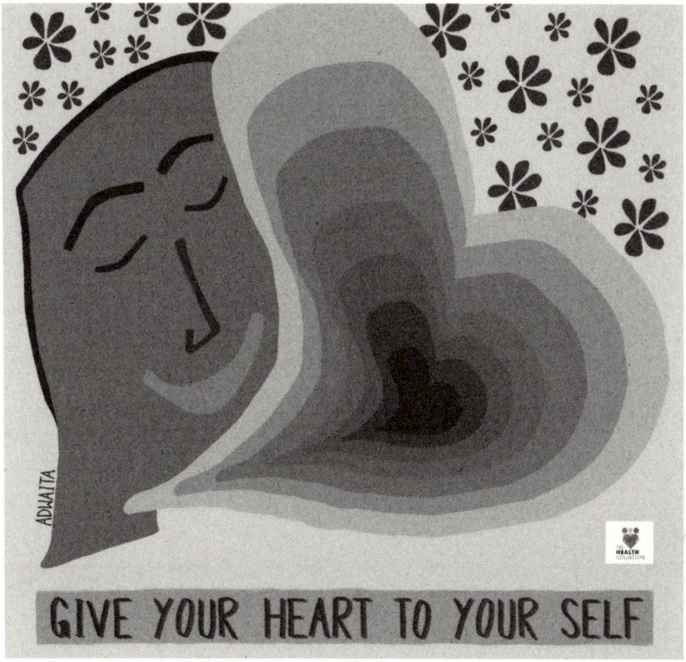

Artist: Adwaita Das

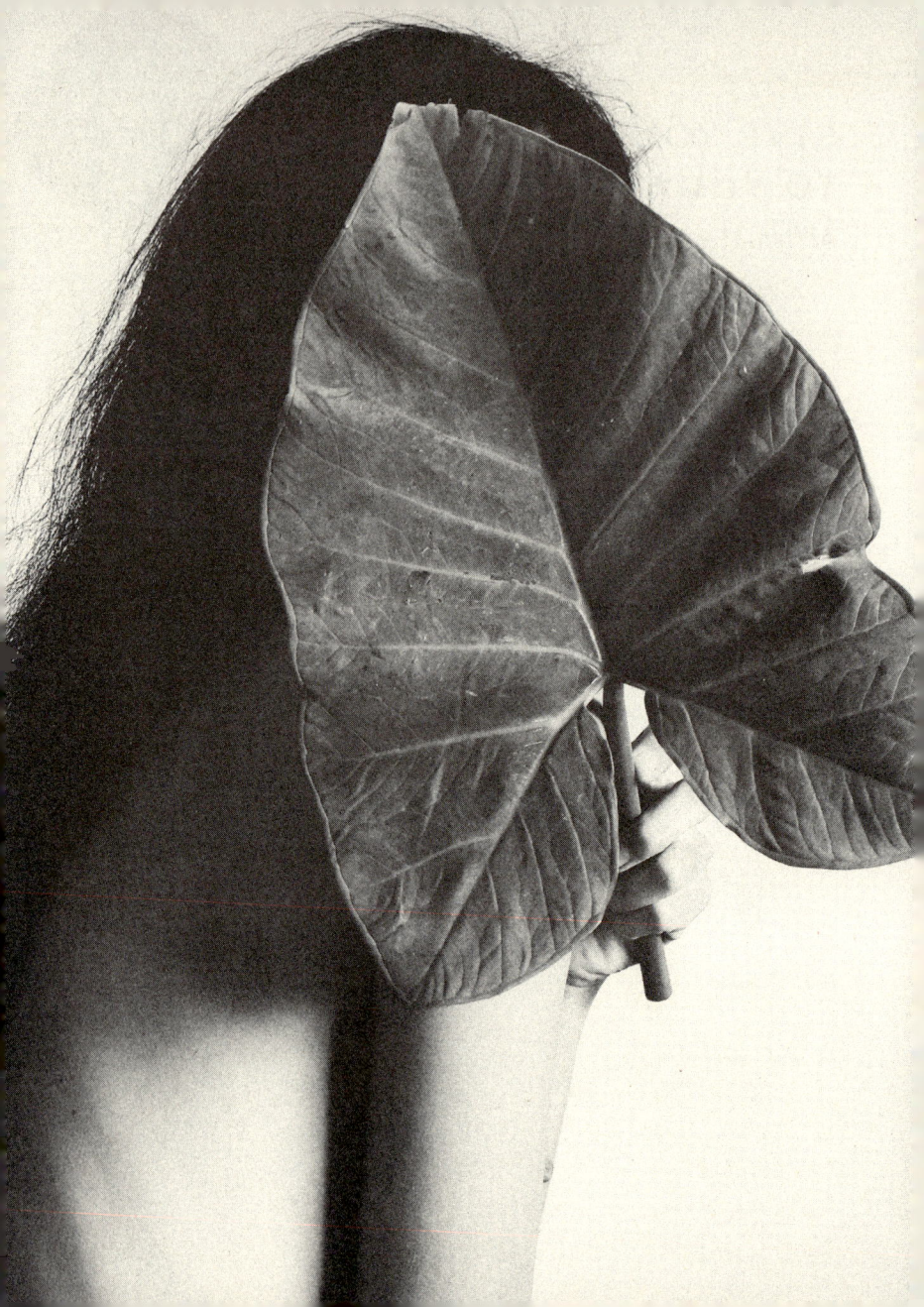

Chapter 8
IN THEIR OWN WORDS
By Manisha Chachra

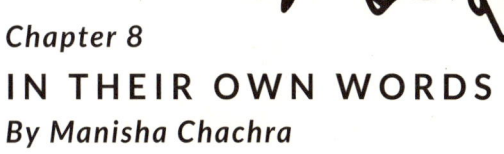

Manisha Chachra is pursuing a PhD in Political Studies from Jawaharlal Nehru University. Her interest areas include sexuality, gender, mental health, Indian politics and hindutva. Manisha shared a very moving[26] first person story with The Health Collective which she has kindly developed further to share more of her journey with you, readers of this book.
She tweets @ChachraManisha

(Trigger warning: Suicidal ideation)

Editor's Note: If you or anyone you know is experiencing extreme thoughts please do reach out to a trained professional for help. Some third-party India-based helplines are listed at the end of this book.

'I want to jump of a cliff,' I messaged my friend when I got off at Tilak Nagar, my home station. He kept talking to me till I reached home and comforted me by simply listening to me. I realised what I was experiencing didn't happen in a day, it had bottled up with time. There was a pivotal need to take help from a mental health professional so that I could look at things objectively. However, before I could come to a decision of finally going for therapy, a pandemonium of opinions gripped my mind.

A lot of friends dismissed my narrative, saying, 'Think about your family,' or *'Chal be! Ek exam nai hua toh, mar jayegi?!'* (*Come on, man, just because one exam hasn't happened, will you die?*)

I've learned first-hand that suicidal stigma leads to avoidance on the part of family and friends to engage with the person having suicidal tendencies.

Garima Garg, a clinical psychologist based in New Delhi, tells The Health Collective, 'As a society we feel threatened whenever anyone complains (about) having suicidal tendencies. At large, everyone wants to immediately fix the issue because they are fearful *ki arey yaar yeh toh marne ki baat kar raha/rahi hai.'* (*Gosh, this person is talking about killing themselves.*)

As a mental health professional Garg says, 'Clients having suicidal tendencies often complain that nobody takes them seriously and if taken seriously they are told to have positive thoughts or go for some spiritual solutions.' In the end, patients either end up feeling 'dejected' or 'suppress emotions to hide the pain.'

It is important to know that professional help is available. Geetika Kapoor, a school psychologist who runs the community outreach initiative EdEssential,

tells The Health Collective, 'A mental health professional is trained to be non-discriminatory and rather understand the client's concern empathetically.'

'It is necessary to have a support system where even laypersons can communicate and understand each other compassionately,' Kapoor adds.

'Thoughts about suicide may have their roots in an underlying mental state which are distressing for the individual. Therefore the management should entail addressing both of these,' says Vikasni Kannan, another psychologist based in New Delhi. 'Along with timely treatment from mental health professionals, enhancing coping skills and building a support system is essential in such cases. The mere knowledge of the fact that there is someone around can help in reducing the distress. As a society, it is crucial that we do not pathologise suicide, and rather try to identify and understand the red flags so that timely help can be provided,' she tells The Health Collective.

The thought of killing oneself 'is a distraction from emotional pain and shifts the focus towards bodily pain,' says Garg. The primary thought is not to 'kill the body'; instead it is to 'end the pain.'

'Families need to emerge as supportive and compassionate units for the patient... In such a vulnerable state, they must be heard out as much as possible,' Garg adds.

It is important to understand that suicidal thoughts do not happen in a day, or just overnight — such thoughts progress over time. A research study[27] conducted in 2017 by Indiaspend indicates that every hour a student commits a suicide in India.

Every hour.

In India, given a dearth of resources (eg a shortage of 87% mental health professionals till 2016, according to this report[28]), it's not enough to just hope that we have enough trained mental health experts on hand.

Editor's Note: If you or anyone you know is feeling vulnerable or suicidal, or at-risk, please do reach out for help. Some third-party helplines are listed on: http://www.healthcollective.in/suicide-prevention-helplines/

We also need to ensure viable support systems. 'There is a need to create a support system that prevents suicide and not just intervene during a crisis,' says Kapoor.

We especially require a focus on preventive measures, given that the invisibility of emotional pain makes it difficult for anyone to seek help and voice it. 'In terms of policy imperatives, mental health professionals need to work at the prevention level. The intervention takes place only when issues go out of control and there is a mental breakdown.'

Kapoor argues: 'A support system needs to be there to make sure that help reaches to at-risk groups in time.'

Other important measures are, 'to introduce (some sort of) emotional training that helps us distinguish between our emotions... How different situations trigger different emotions. For instance often embarrassment is confused with anger, hurt is confused with irritation, etc.'

Furthermore, it is necessary to increase conversations in real life, face-to-face, she emphasises, rather than on screens. 'If five kids are sitting together in a room and are engaged in their phones, there is no eye contact: I see that as a dangerous situation because these kids will never get an opportunity to develop communication skills,' Kapoor warns.

As someone who experiences suicidal thoughts every now and then because rough phases don't get over in a jiffy, I have learned that talking it out is the key.

It is crucial to have fellow comrades in whom one can confide. The incessant talking on the phone and meeting new people helps immensely in lightening the burden of our hearts. However, professional help reconciled the differences between my rationality and emotions. Therapy has enabled me to cope with these emotions such that I accept hurt without being negative.

Garg says, 'In a situation when you feel suicidal, it is important to share your concern with someone you can completely trust ... It is only when (the) suicidal feeling intensifies that a person is forced to take an adverse step, most of the times clients are desperately looking for someone to talk to.'

Similarly, Kapoor says, 'as friends we must ask one another how are they doing? Call up our friends frequently, and keep human interaction alive. Merely knowing someone is there to check on us can build trust among one another.'

...

This episode was a crucial turning point for multiple realisations about my mental health. The most important one is that I needed support and therapy for a longer period of time. In my therapy sessions, I comprehended that suicidal ideations do not happen out of the blue. They are a result of bottled up emotions that need a slow and steady release.

A therapeutic environment ensures trust and empathy, which was majorly lacking in my relationships. My anxieties and feelings found a comfortable abode in my therapist's proactive reception of my emotions.

With my thoughts of suicidal ideation, I realised how imperative it is to have an ally, and to have healthy relationships in our lives. As therapy was going on, I opened up in my conversations with friends and family about my feelings and vulnerabilities. You know you have great and healthy relationships when you can be vulnerable and honest with others. It made me understand that authentic friendships allow for a space to be vulnerable and stay true to who we are.

Initially, therapy is challenging, as you may confront shattering of worlds and realms within you — realms of your imagination, fears, and vulnerabilities. However, healing happens when we begin to trust ourselves and our therapist in the process. You will know that you are mentally growing and coping up better with the storms of life when you are aware of what is going on.

My therapist repeatedly reminded me that even if you are aware, you will be able to let your feelings be and get 'unstuck', yourself.

Therapy has been a voyage in developing skills for my mental health. Skills like resilience, which has been the most important one here, aiding me in having honest conversations with myself. Within a year, in my sessions, I realised therapy is an investment that every adult should be motivated to make. My family was (initially) not very open to the idea of seeking professional help, but now I can have a dialogue with them about its significant contribution to my mental growth.

For anyone going through hard days even in therapy, I would like to tell you that some days are all sweat and toil, but growth will feel like a victory. Healing never happens in a day and it varies from person to person — the only way out is letting out how you feel — as often and as honestly as we can.

One piece of advice from me? Let people who are suffering know they are not alone.

SUICIDE PREVENTION: CREATING THE SPACE TO SEEK HELP[29]
By Kamna Chhibber

This piece originally appeared on The Health Collective.

Speaking, talking and sharing are not always given space in society. Often we shy away from discussing difficult issues. We find it a challenge to share our true thoughts and feelings. Many feel that what goes on within them may not be acceptable to others around them and in society at large. A perception develops whereby we start dictating our communications to conform to certain set standards and norms.

The more we see that certain types of communication do not occur in our social fabric, the more we withdraw within our own self. The need to share gets associated with a feeling of weakness and a questioning of the strength of the self-system to handle and deal with problems. It continuously and in a vicious way impacts self-concepts, relationships and our adjustment to the environment in which we exist.

And yet, increasingly we are surrounded by situations where people are breaking the norm. This happens when collectively, we as a community and a society, come together to challenge existing belief systems and ways of doing things. Getting ourselves together is not an easy task but it is not impossible. Generating awareness and understanding of the need for the desired change is the first step in moving towards breaking existing norms. One norm that we most certainly need to break is that of silence that surrounds mental health and its vicissitudes. A move to break the shackles that bind people from disclosing and talking about what affects them, their moods, thinking, situations, experiences and mental health conditions is a must in society today.

Discourse around mental health challenges needs to become a norm instead of the silence that currently permeates it and this can start by encouraging people to talk, share and seek help when they need it.

Know when someone needs help: The same situation can have a different impact on individuals. Our standards for ourselves find no application as a determining factor as to who may or may not need help. The most important aspect which indicates that help is needed by an individual is their subjective level of distress on account of any situation.

Distress which continues to exist despite time and situation changing or support being available is an indicator of a situation which warrants seeking help. When an individual's functionality is affected, their ways of doing things at their workplace, home and social spaces is impacted, it is a red flag that necessitates giving a deeper look to what is going on with the individual.

Verbalisations by an individual of finding it difficult to cope with situations or of an internal struggle that does not seem to abate, make it a must that one encourage the person to seek help for what they are struggling with.

Directing someone to the help they need: It is not easy to go up to someone and simply state *'I think you need help, so go meet an expert'*. It can come across as harsh, presumptuous or derogatory to the individual. There are some things to be kept in mind to enable help seeking in an individual:

- Every individual has their own sensitivities and encouraging someone to seek help requires you to be cognizant of these so you can be empathetic in your approach to the person
- It helps to share your understanding of how difficult the current experiences may be for the individual. This creates a space for you to have a conversation before you can direct them to professional help
- Express your care and concern without being too dramatic or emotional in your discourse and narrative. Sticking to facts, specifically to your own observations, is most helpful in such a situation
- Share your availability to the individual and also possibility of your presence when they decide to make their first phone call to an expert or visit to an expert. It can be comforting for the person to know that there is support available for them
- Ensure you have your information in place with details of helplines or experts who the person can reach out to for help
- Be sure to mention that seeking help is not a sign of weakness or lack of strength and ability in the individual. It is like visiting a doctor for a physical ailment and no different. Busting these myths and ideas can be comforting for the person and can go a long way in ensuring that they do seek help at the earliest
- Most importantly, continue to stay connected even post the initial contact for seeking help by the individual. Your support is going to be irreplaceable even as experts work with the person

It's important to emphasise:

Help-seeking is in no way a sign of a deficit. It takes courage to step outside, acknowledge that you have a problem, recognise that you may not be able to find a solution and speak to experts who are nevertheless strangers about all that goes on within you. There are various helplines that are available where you can speak

about what is going on.

Please do reach out if you or a loved one feels like you need help.

Find the right expert for yourself and don't hesitate even if you need to go through a few people before you feel comfortable in working with someone. There are certain questions you can answer for yourself to decide if your therapist/expert is right for you. You can read more on that on The Health Collective[30].

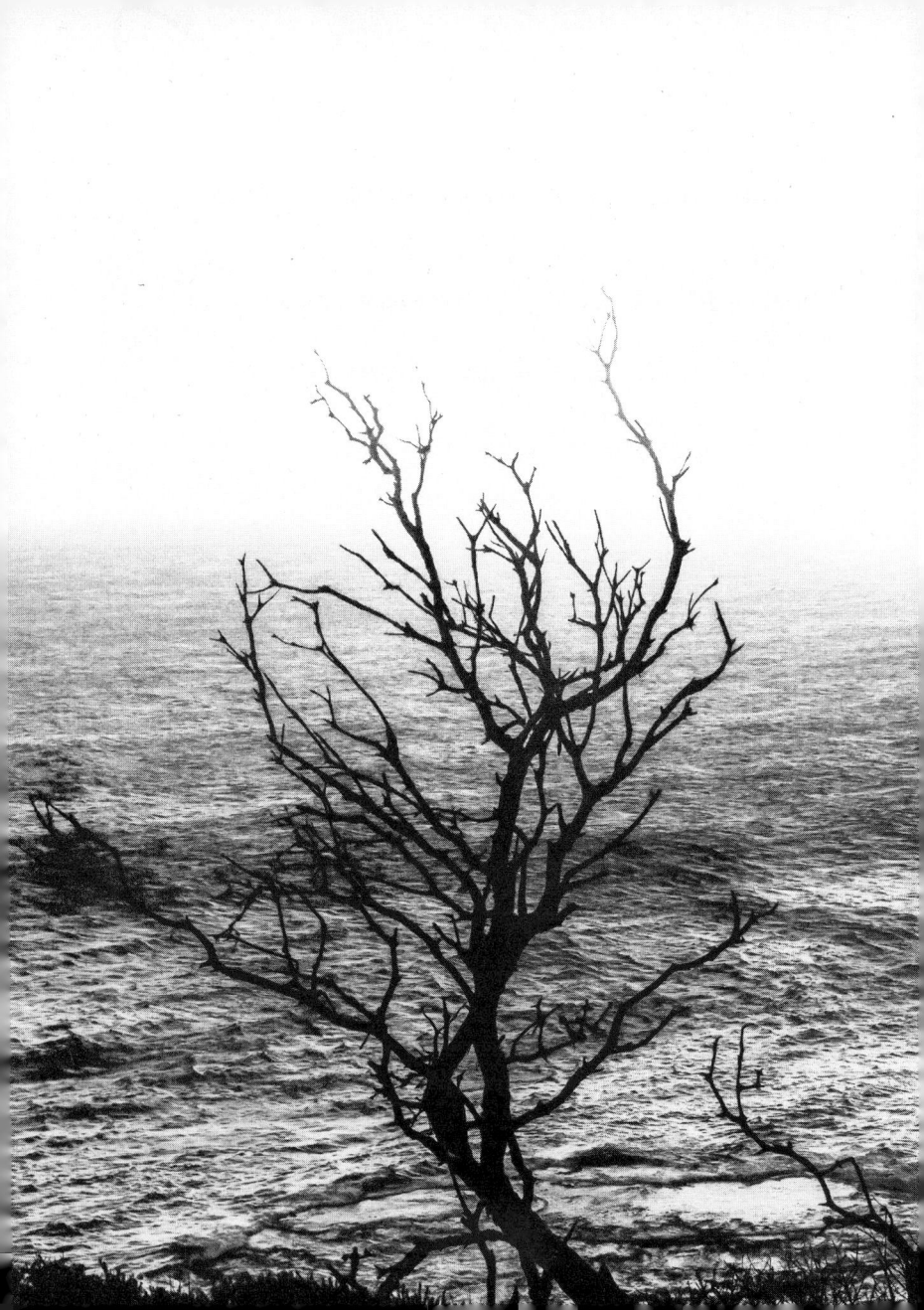

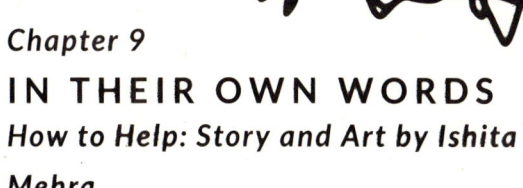

Chapter 9
IN THEIR OWN WORDS
How to Help: Story and Art by Ishita Mehra

About the Artist: Ishita Mehra is a young mental health advocate and illustrator. Her work includes writing and illustrating personal stories of people about their mental health struggles, illustrating mental health themes and subjects and initiating workshops on mental health. Currently, she is focusing on starting a support group in Pune to allow people to access and facilities on mental health care. You can find her on Instagram @VoiletHill.

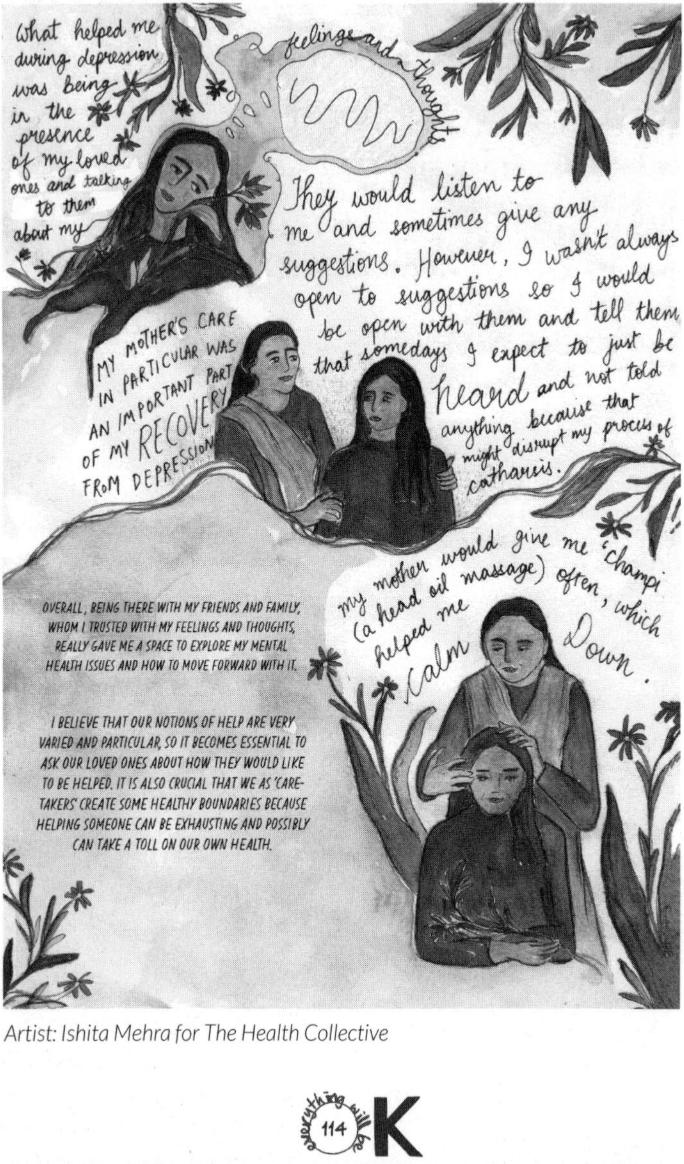

Young MENTAL HEALTH

Artist: Ishita Mehra for The Health Collective

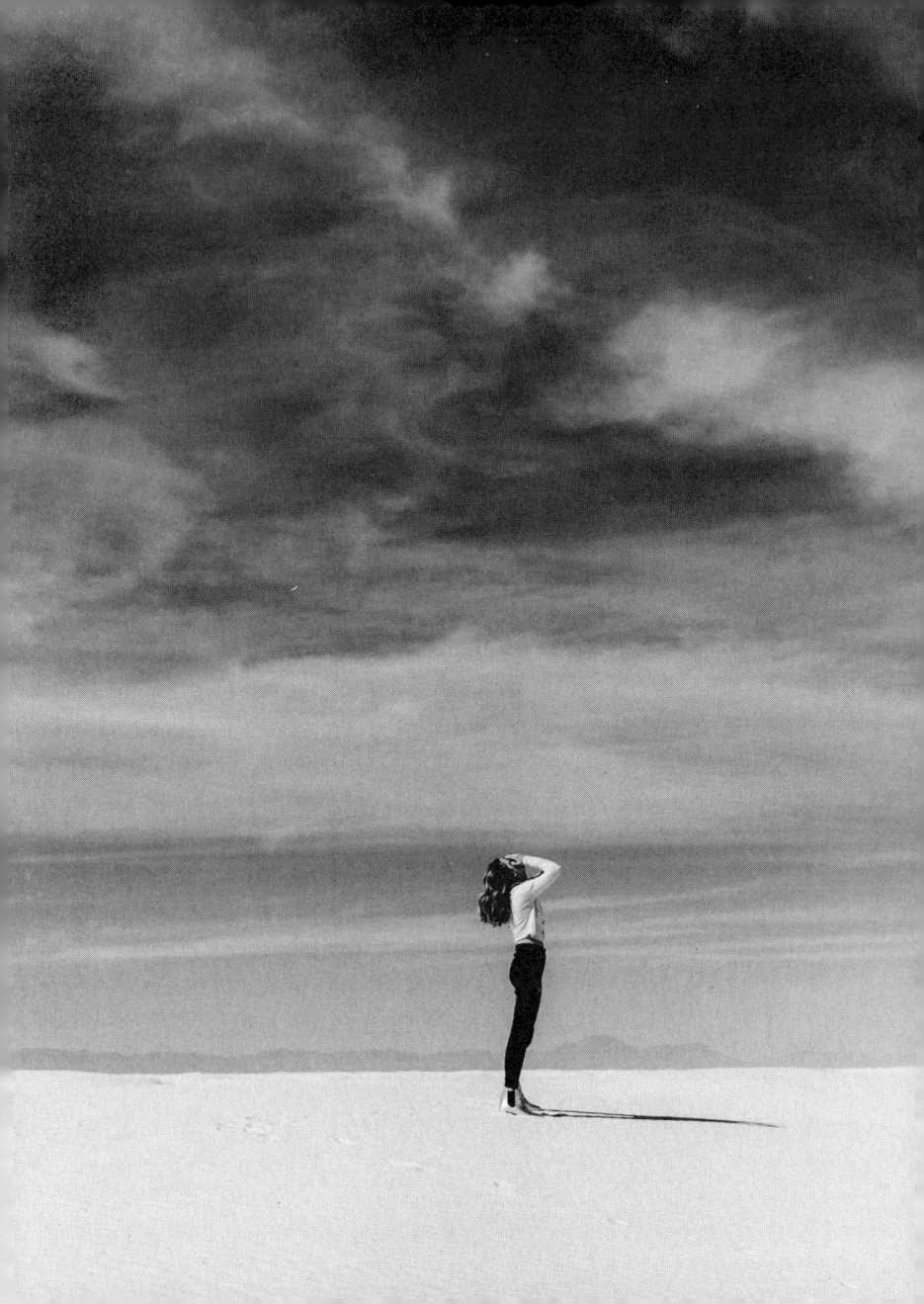

Chapter 10
IN THEIR OWN WORDS: YOUTH SPEAK

What do students have to say for themselves? Mohit Dhingra, an alumnus of the Young India Fellowship, a theatre artiste, spoken word poet and street photographer is passionate about India's need to set up a 24x7 mental health emergency helpline. He shared some of the findings of a small survey (of ~300 students) with The Health Collective website conducted at a leading university in India:

'A small survey taken at one of India's leading universities found some astounding results. Anxiety attacks and panic attacks, negative reaction to substances, suicidal thoughts, inability to focus and carry out daily chores and self-harm were some of the major categories of issues that people considered as a mental health emergency. 73% of those surveyed had either experienced or encountered a mental health emergency in the past. On facing such an emergency, 64% of respondents chose to reach out to their friends for help, 32% resorted to professionals while a staggering 67% decided to handle it by themselves.

On the other hand, a meagre 3.7% decided to reach out to a mental health emergency helpline. When asked if a helpline of such nature would be helpful in dealing with mental health emergencies, help de-escalate them effectively and if their university needed one, over 91% of people answered yes. *(While this survey was done on a small sample size of ~300 university students, the results are quite eye-opening.)*' [31]

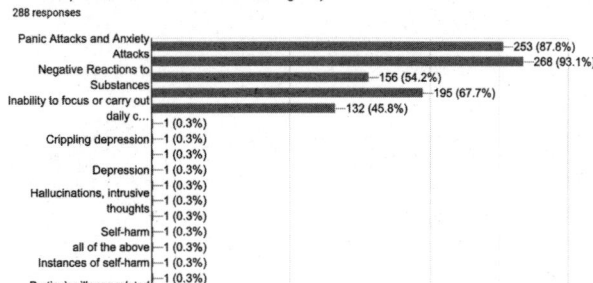

Courtesy: Mohit Dhingra

Have you ever encountered or experienced a Mental Health Emergency?

288 responses

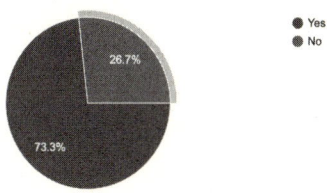

- Yes 73.3%
- No 26.7%

If you've had a Mental Health Emergency, where or whom did you reach out to?

242 responses

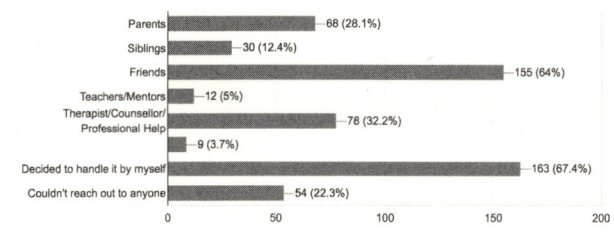

- Parents — 68 (28.1%)
- Siblings — 30 (12.4%)
- Friends — 155 (64%)
- Teachers/Mentors — 12 (5%)
- Therapist/Counsellor/Professional Help — 78 (32.2%)
- — 9 (3.7%)
- Decided to handle it by myself — 163 (67.4%)
- Couldn't reach out to anyone — 54 (22.3%)

YOUTHBOL SURVEY: WHAT'S THE HEALTH WISHLIST FOR ONE LAKH YOUNG INDIANS?

YouthBol, a campaign launched last September by the Centre for Catalysing Change and its partner USAID's Maternal Child Survival Plan Project, released findings from a poll that reached more than one lakh young Indians. The idea was to find out what Young India's priorities are when it comes to health and well-being.

Their press release specifies that the poll reached out to 1,10,092 people across three age groups (10–14, 15–9 and 20–24) in 27 states and four union territories, via field as well as online outreach.

Key findings, quoting from their press release:

- In percentage terms, 10–24 year olds in India — indicate the YouthBol results — have two key concerns that preoccupy them: health and in-school services. Thirty-six per cent of the over one lakh respondents said health was their top priority, while 26 per cent laid emphasis on in-school facilities.
- Under the broad category of health-related responses, the most strident demand that YouthBol has thrown up has been for information (and action) on prevention of substance abuse.
- Many young women polled by YouthBol ranked access to information and care on menstruation, menstrual pain management, and menstrual hygiene and products at the top of their wish-list.
- For the oldest age group (20–24 years), information on and access to contraceptive methods and family planning services emerged as a key priority. This demand was also the highest among YouthBol respondents who were married.
- Mental health-related information and services is also a priority theme.

YouthBol indicates that young people want information on how to cope with academic pressure and stress, peer-pressure and bullying. They also want better access to non-judgemental, confidential, and affordable mental health services.

- For young people who stated they were in relationships, obtaining more information on sexual attraction, love and relationships emerged as a strong priority. [32]

IN THEIR OWN WORDS: YOUTH MENTAL HEALTH ADVOCATE ANANYA DHANUKA

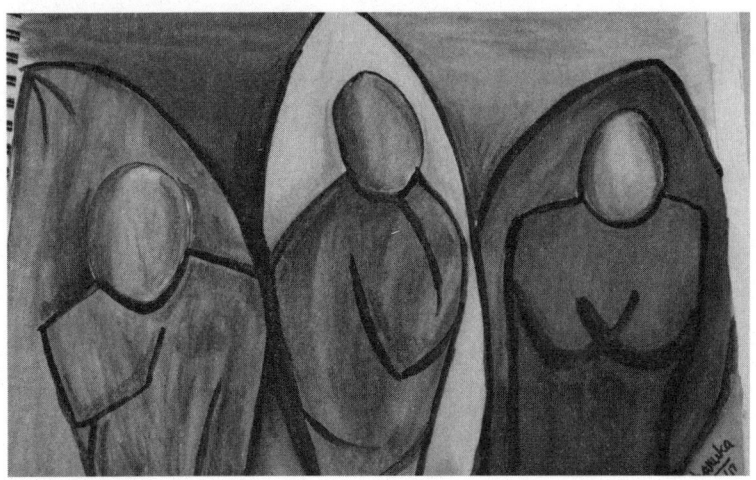

Image courtesy Ananya Dhanuka

THE THREE PLAYERS
Republished with permission from Ananya Dhanuka [33]

They call me names, punch my face, push me away. They act like I don't exist. Why do they do this?

Why me? The one feeling that every bullied person experiences. And there's really no answer for it. But there is a solution — to act whenever you see an event take place. To take action and report to teachers, seniors, officials, anyone who can help you.

When such a situation occurs, there are three actors in play: the bully, the bullied and the bystander.

- The bully is the one who takes aggressive action against the bullied, for his own reasons.
- The bullied is the sufferer of social isolation, verbal and physical abuse. The bullied is encouraged to stand up, to speak for themselves. To not let other people overpower them.
- The bystander. Those who witness these acts play the most crucial role in helping us curb bullying. They have the power to intervene, to take action and create an intolerant environment towards bullying.
- It is essential to analyse these players because they help us arise (sic) at the root cause of the issue. It educates us about the need to become more aware, vigilant and sensitive (of) our environments.

I'm a mind-speaker, you can be too.

Ananya Dhanuka is a 17-year-old student finishing up with Class XII in New Delhi. She has been part of an anti-bullying programme with the Fortis Mental Young Mental Health Advocates, which we will read more about in the second part of this book. She shares her experience, her blog post on bullying here, and why she thinks we all need to talk more and stop taking our mental health so casually.

Young
MENTAL HEALTH

ANANYA DHANUKA: I'm 17 years old. I've been in the same school for the last 14 years, which practically means I've been in the same school all my life. I've always been aware of my environment, social in my gatherings and not afraid to vocalise issues.

AMRITA: What led to your interest in learning about mental health?

ANANYA DHANUKA: I've been very active and social in school, taking up leadership roles in the student council for the last three years. As I took these positions, the more I started realising the issues that our school faced, starting with the grim state of emphasis we put on the mental health of our students. This was coupled with the Fortis Bully to Buddy campaign in our school. I was made in-charge of the project, which gave me further insight and deeper understanding of the impact that bullying has on school students, especially given the new age peer and parental pressure.

AMRITA: Can you describe what the Youth Mental Health Advocate programme has been like? What has your experience been like? Did you enjoy it? What can you share about the anti-bullying programme?

ANANYA DHANUKA: The Young Mental Health Advocate Programme has been one of the greatest learning experiences in my high school years. It gave me exposure to psychology, greater sensitivity to mental health problems and empowered me to become of assistance to those around me. The opportunity to interact with specialists in the field of psychology and journalism taught me how to influence my environment to bring about a mental revolution, the need of the hour. Along with that, I met amazing fellow advocates who are in college or in school, which brought a lot of personal experiences and knowledge to the table. I enjoyed every meeting I was a part of because I felt like I was finally contributing to society, and improving myself personally as well.

The anti-bullying programme consisted of proper training from the Fortis hospital, for students who were selected to the Anti-bullying Squad formed in our school. The anti-bullying programme has been the most meaningful experience I've had.

AMRITA: What was the biggest take-away?

ANANYA DHANUKA: My biggest takeaway has been understanding the influence of minute actions on people and their emotions. It made me realise how casually we take mental health, often not even deeming it worthy of attention.

AMRITA: How easy or difficult is it to talk to peers or friends and family about issues to do with mental health and mental illness?

ANANYA DHANUKA: I feel like even though our generation is becoming increasingly aware about mental health issues and the need to be sensitive, yet it is still ignored or taken as a weakness. I've personally felt it, considering it to be 'stupid' since they were just 'joking' and didn't mean harm. It does become difficult to make people realise their mistakes if they don't agree that the problem exists in the first place.

I think the same holds with family. Even though parents do talk to their children these days, mental health issues are firstly, tough to open up about, secondly, rubbed off as general stress or a 'phase'.

AMRITA: Did you think that folks at your high school were open in talking about mental health? What made it easier or harder to have these conversations?

ANANYA DHANUKA: I feel like the people in my school are interested and desperately need someone to talk to, about their issues. However, they are afraid to talk to each other about it. They still dread being judged for having problems. The taboo still persists.

AMRITA: Do you think that bullying is something that is quite common? Any examples/anecdotes you can share?

ANANYA DHANUKA: I do feel it is quite common. I also feel like saying bullying only exists in schools or offices is restricting the meaning of bullying. It can happen in any environment, it is a huge prevailing problem, and the most ignored of all. I would say the most prominent example I can think of is cyber-bullying. Being targeted, virtually harassed, made memes of. It's uncontrollable and impacts you directly.

AMRITA: What does your family think of your interest in

mental health/illness and do you find it easy to have these conversations at home?

ANANYA DHANUKA: My parents have always been supportive when it came to my work. Luckily they have been open to listening to my problems. Although naturally, sometimes conflicts do arise when they fail to understand the problem from my point of view, as a teenager struggling with significant life changes.

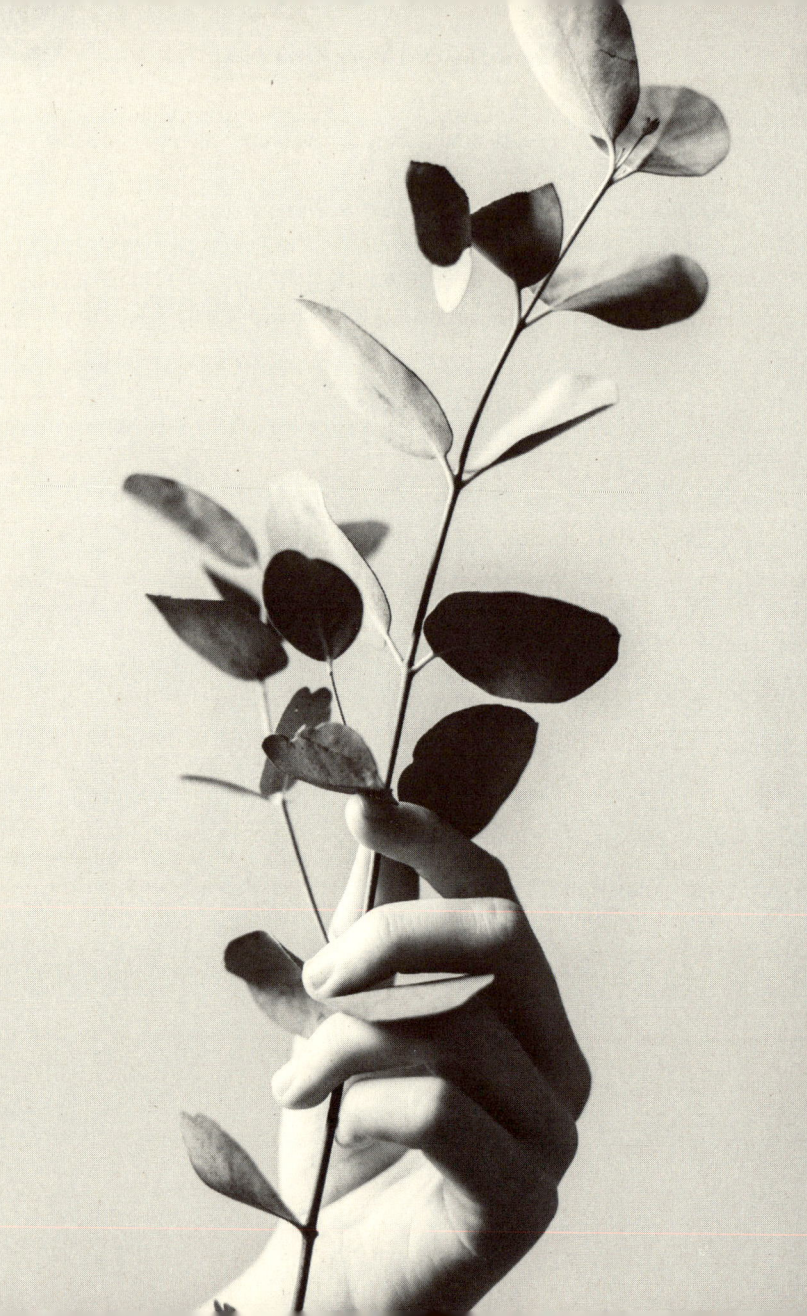

Chapter 11
IN THEIR OWN WORDS
COULD THIS BE HOME?
Art and Words by Solo

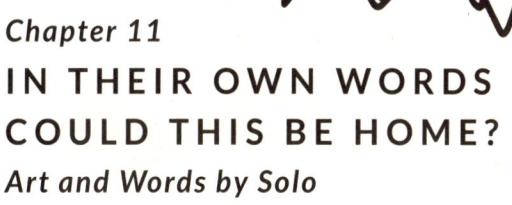

About the Artist: Solo is a writer and cartoonist from Bangalore. She likes reading, playing video games and binge-watching Netflix. Her life would have been rather unremarkable had it not been for her BPD-fuelled imagination. She also has four cats. Check out more work at stripteasethemag.com

Young
MENTAL HEALTH

COULD THIS BE HOME?

BY SOLO

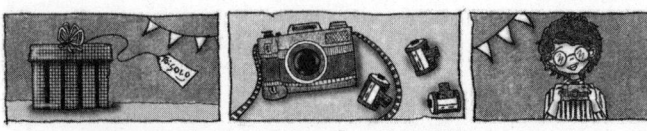

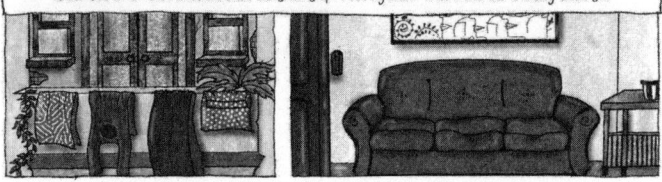

It was around 1998 when I realised that I was growing up in a family where mental illness wasn't exactly a stranger.

I hated it. I hated it so much. Being called the Addams Family wasn't as pride inducing as it is now.

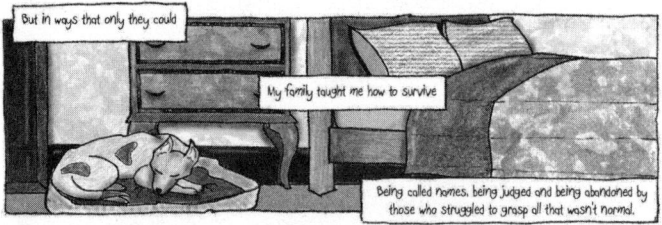

But in ways that only they could

My family taught me how to survive

Being called names, being judged and being abandoned by those who struggled to grasp all that wasn't normal.

They taught me to hate myself less and they taught me to take pride in the fact that I wasn't like the rest. The fact that I could never be.

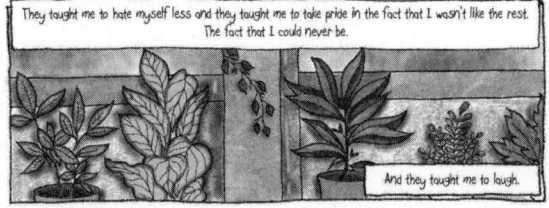

And they taught me to laugh.

I learned to laugh at being ridiculously different, and to embrace the beauty of absurdity, the power of imagination and the freedom that comes with it.

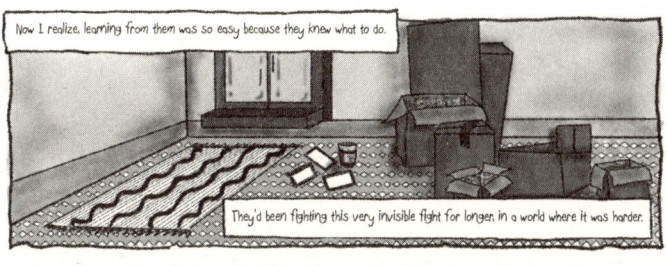

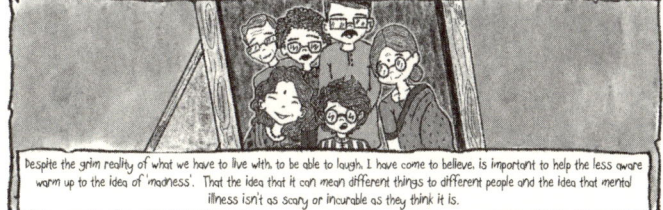

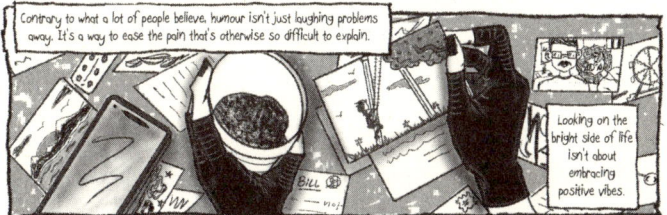

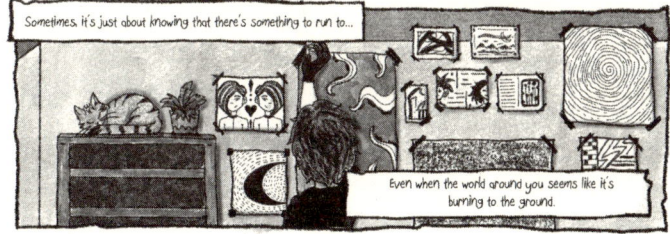

I ACCEPT DEEP, RESTFUL, PEACEFUL SLEEP

Affirmation by Adwaita Das

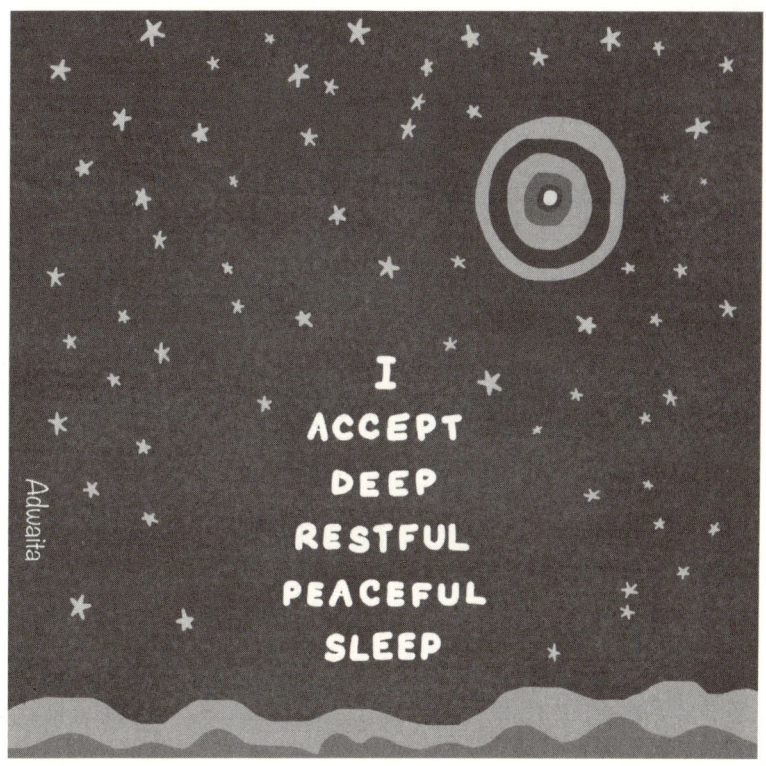

Artist: Adwaita Das

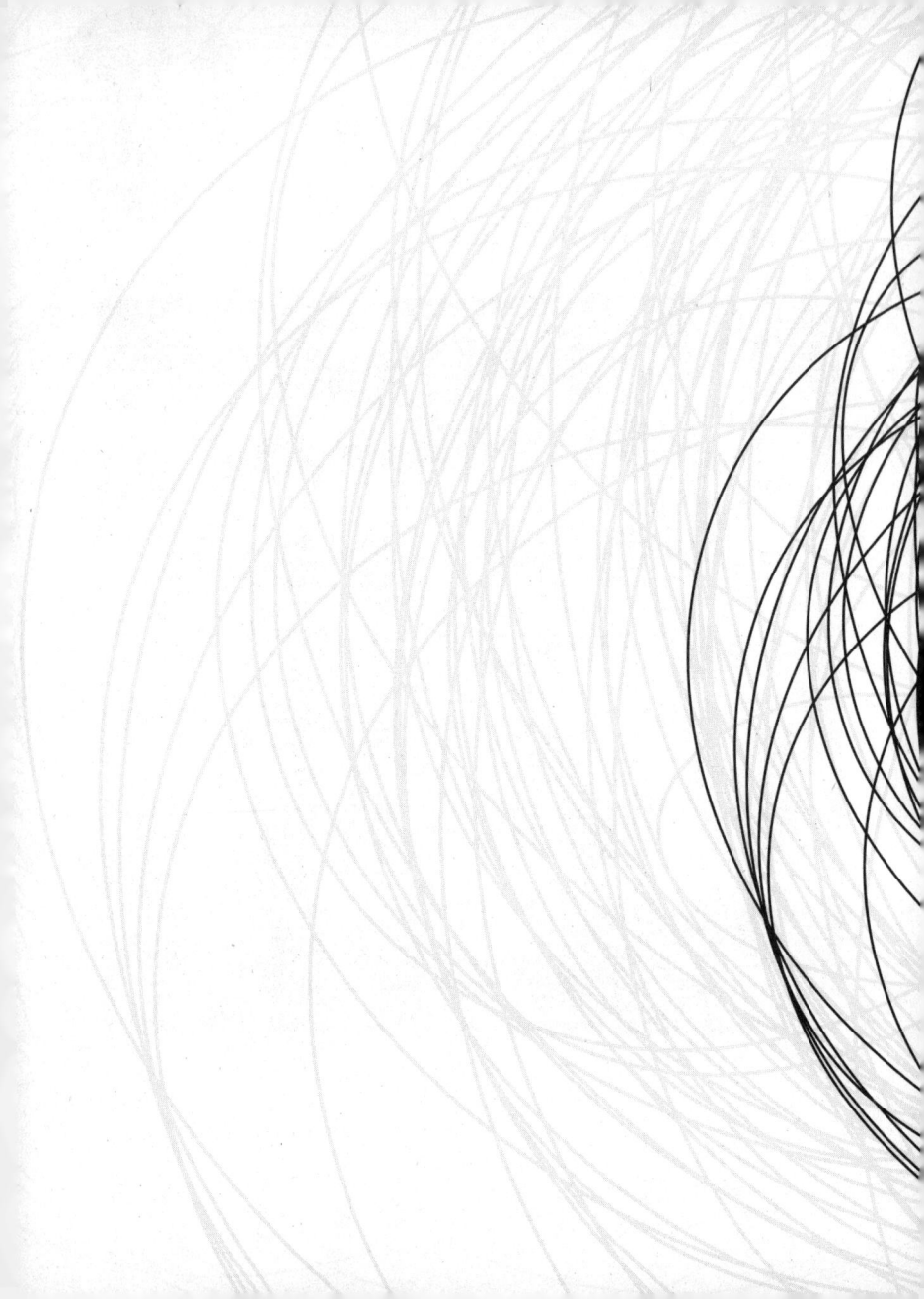

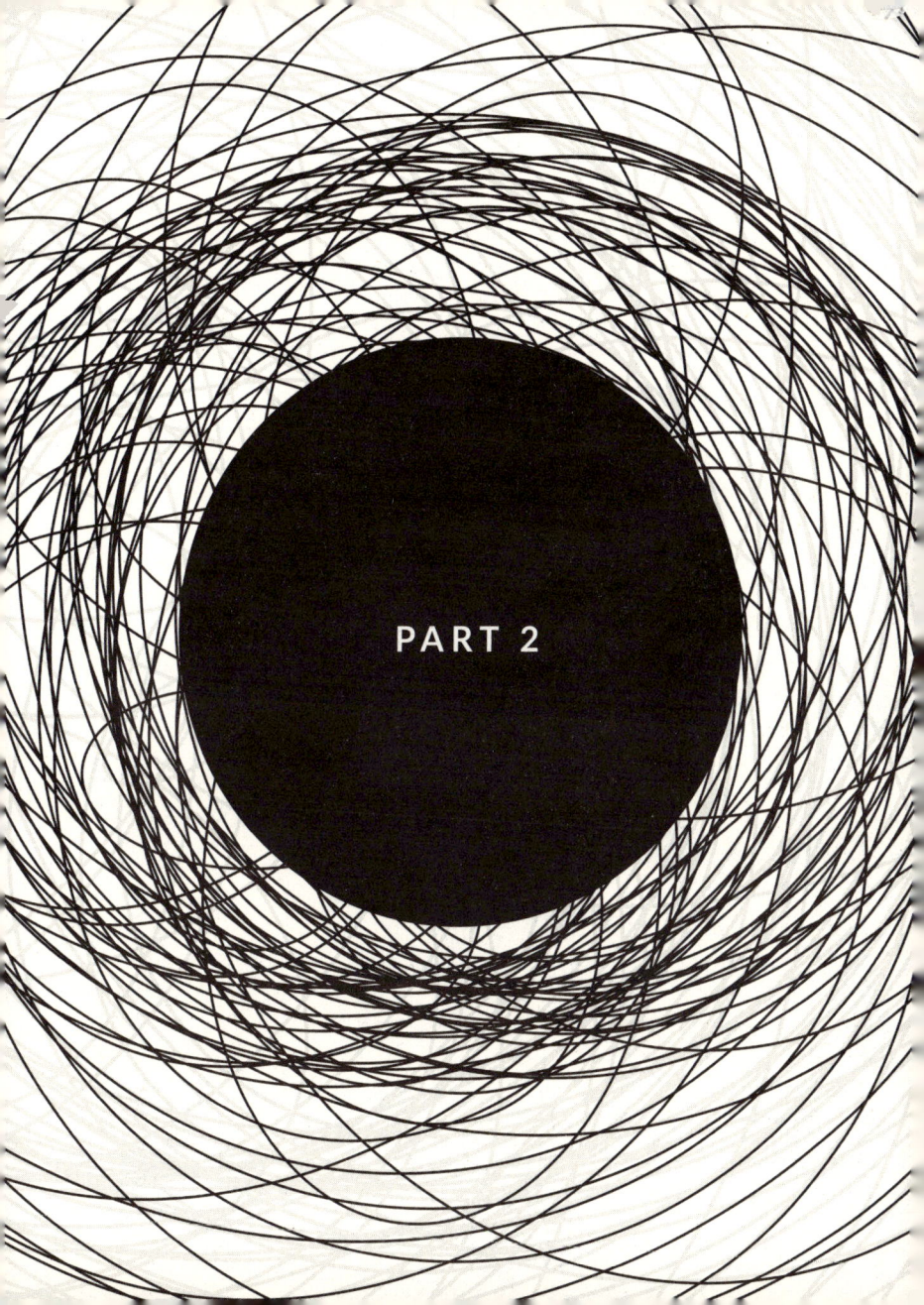

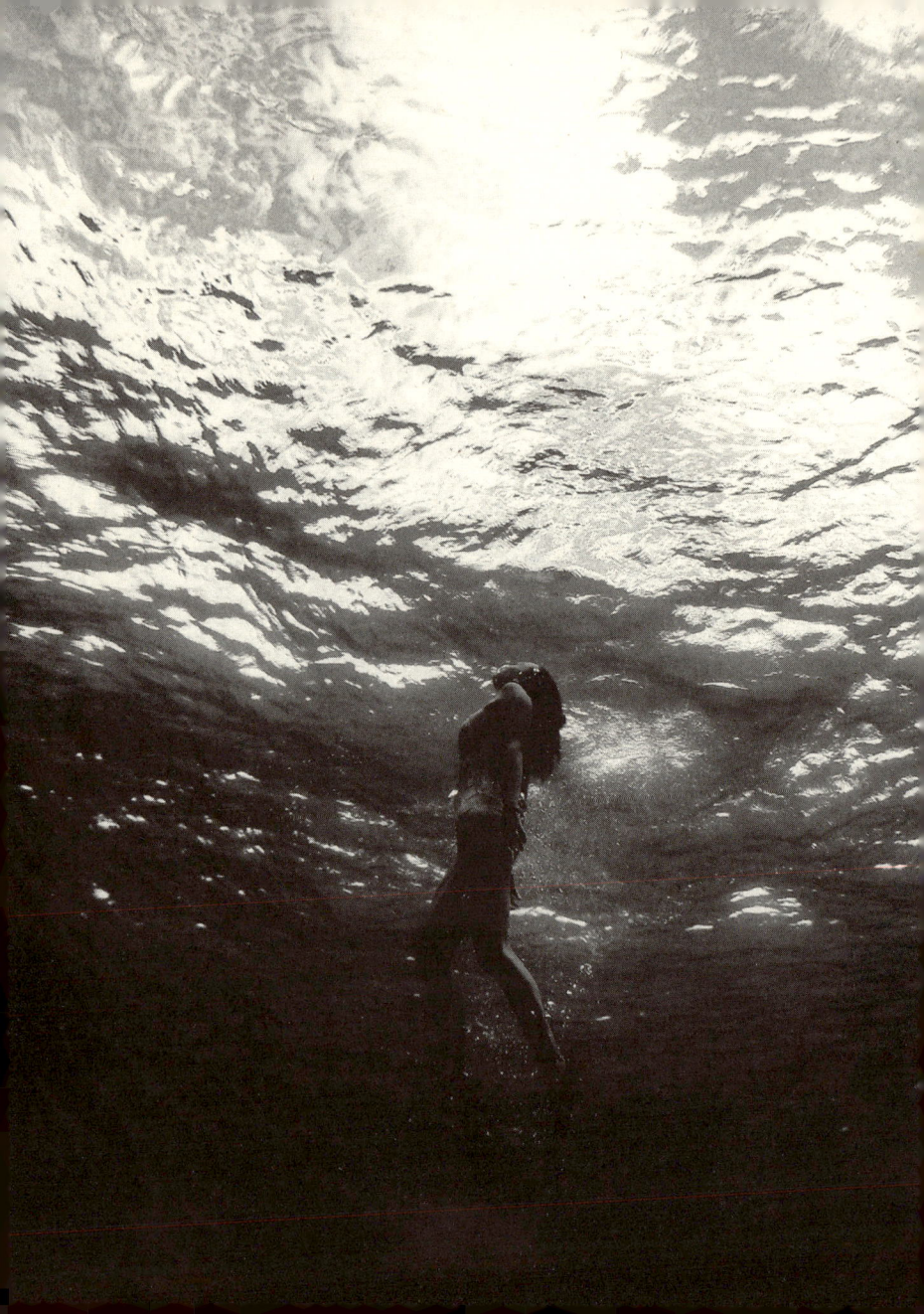

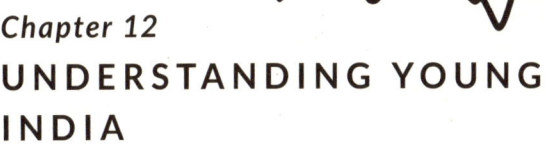

Chapter 12
UNDERSTANDING YOUNG INDIA

Apart from anecdotal examples and cyclical media coverage on 'exam stress', how do we begin to unpack young India's mental health experience? Through their own words and analysis of work being done by counsellors, some key themes emerge. A recent paper published on the peer-reviewed medical journal *BMJ Open* shared key findings from a content analysis of what young Indians were saying about mental health. The paper (Gonsalves P et al)[34] looked at 37 submissions by 33 authors between the ages of 19 to 31 from seven cities, and found multiple themes in the submissions.

Four themes were identified:

- Living through difficulties
- Mental health in context
- Managing one's mental health
- Breaking stigma and sharing hope

Overall, the participants expressed significant feelings of distress and hopelessness as a result of their mental health problems; many described the context of their difficulties as resulting from personal histories or wider societal factors; a general lack of understanding about mental health; and widespread stigma and other negative attitudes. Most participants expressed a desire to overcome mental health prejudice and discrimination.'

For more information, we spoke to Pattie Gonsalves, author of the paper cited above, who works as a Project Director with the NGO Sangath and leads the anti-stigma programmes *It's Ok to Talk* and *Mann Mela*, which focus on youth outreach.

The website itsoktotalk.in describes itself as 'a safe space to share your experiences with mental health, mental illness and well-being. We believe that talking about mental health is the first step to breaking the stigma.'[35]

Pattie is also one of the directors of the PRIDE adolescent research programme, which is creating a smartphone game[36] that helps adolescents learn problem-solving skills and improve their mental health. Here are lightly edited excerpts from our interview.

AMRITA: How many young people would you estimate you have worked with at It's Ok to Talk since the site was launched on World Mental Health Day in 2017? Can you set the context by sharing more about this work?

PATTIE GONSALVES: Over the past three years, 2.5 million via social media; 7,000+ directly through events and workshops; 280 volunteers; 50 youth advocates have been trained in mental health leadership.

In sharing our stories with others, we find comfort, strength, hope, and often, solidarity. While the circumstances, timelines and details may differ, the stories of our dreams, desires, relationships and struggles, invariably coincide. Every individual travels a unique journey through their experiences. Few seem to cope better than others, some have regular ups and downs, thriving at times and struggling otherwise, and yet others appear to struggle all the time. At It's Ok To Talk, we believe that mental health is one of our most important human assets, and it helps us navigate the world around us. Today, a systemic lack of investment in mental health puts us in a serious mental health crisis. Solving this complex challenge through building awareness about mental health is at the heart of our work.

India has the world's largest population of young people (ages 10–24)[37], and mental health problems are the leading health concern for this age group. In fact, suicide is a leading cause of death for young Indians.

At the same time, fewer than 10 per cent of young Indians have access to formal mental health services, highlighting an urgent need to identify innovative strategies to promote mental health for this age group nationally. [38]

World over, there is now also a growing interest in the use of various multi-

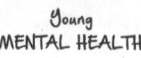
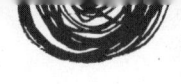

media and social media platforms as vehicles for mental health promotion and stigma reduction at a population level, particularly among young people. Set in this context, the It's Ok To Talk website was set up, taking inspiration from 'Depression: Let's Talk', the WHO theme for World Mental Health Day in 2017 emphasising the importance of personal disclosure. 2017 was significant in that depression and mental health were raised as significant issues on a global 'health' stage (and not just mental health). Our website invites young people to share their personal stories of experiencing mental health needs, resilience and recovery in any media form of their choice.

AMRITA: What are the primary ways in which mental health/mental illness concerns present themselves?

PATTIE GONSALVES: In terms of what we have seen through the website, four over-arching themes have been identified through the narratives shared:

- Living through difficulties
- Mental health in context
- Managing one's mental health
- Breaking stigma and sharing hope

The stories shared offer a window into the experiences of young people's lives, highlighting how they negotiate different challenges, identities, choices and circumstances related to their mental health. We hope that in learning about their

stories, readers will think more deeply about their own mental health and be more sensitive to others around them.

Loneliness, isolation and a strong desire for connection were prominent (mirroring findings from qualitative studies of youth narratives obtained in high-income countries).

Many young contributors described their mental health difficulties within the context of broader socio-economic and cultural contexts. These submissions went beyond the mere description of internal experiences (thoughts and feelings) to explore and challenge the societal and political contexts of psychological distress, offering a rich and multidimensional understanding of mental health.

In particular, young people's narratives explained how rigid social norms can result in oppressive and unrealistic expectations, exacerbating stress and contributing to poor mental health. (This is also consistent with what we see in other parts of the world where academic, interpersonal and family difficulties are among the key social determinants of poor mental health and suicide in young people.)

The influence of stigma was prominent in narratives around recovery, and particularly the finding that acceptance of mental health problems appeared to be a central part of many authors' journeys of recovery. For some young people, expressing themselves and articulating their experience was part of this process. Many contributors expressed personal motivations to mitigate public stigma, to reduce self-stigma and to help others.

Young
MENTAL HEALTH

AMRITA: Can you talk to us about any on-ground projects like Mann Mela, what are the objectives and any findings so far?

PATTIE GONSALVES: Continuing our mission to increase awareness about mental health and reduce stigma through on-ground efforts and the use of (novel) technology, Mann Mela (or 'Festival of the Mind') was launched in 2019. Mann Mela is a traveling museum of interactive projects and artefacts, created using a mix of arts, technology and science to reflect the stories of real individuals' lived experiences with mental health needs, told through the components of the museum.

It is a collaboration between an interdisciplinary team of young people, including those with lived experiences of mental health needs, researchers and experts, designers, artists and technologists and is being implemented in collaboration with Quicksand Design Studio. It is supported by the Wellcome Trust, UK. Mann Mela plans to travel to Bhopal, Goa, Imphal, New Delhi and Mumbai … and will serve as a mental health resource for individuals and organisations.

The exhibits you will see at Mann Mela will be interactive portraits of young individuals. We are designing these through a unique process of identifying and interviewing contributors, identification of themes from their stories, and finally, the co-design and creation of interactive exhibits where the contributor plays a central role.

There is now a growing understanding about more 'immersive' methods (like virtual reality) that allow people to 'step into someone else's shoes' and can help build empathy, self-reflexivity and invite audiences to understand their own misconceptions. We expect that with the ever-increasing use of digital infrastructures, especially by youth, the role of these kinds of digital projects will become even more significant.

AMRITA: What are the most common mental health concerns or issues that come up with young people (with any caveat as to limitations of analysis or outreach)?

PATTIE GONSALVES: On our website and at our events, we frequently receive questions about managing stress, anxiety, depression and suicidal thoughts. We also receive experiences by young people living with serious mental illnesses, but these are less common.

AMRITA: What are some common or more colloquial words used to describe mental health issues in the various states that you and the team (It's Ok to Talk and Sangath) work in?

PATTIE GONSALVES: 'Tension' is one of the most commonly used words to describe stress and mental health problems. I think this also speaks about the culture/context of the language (i.e., limited vocabulary) we have to describe our thoughts, feelings and behaviours (i.e., what makes up our 'mental health') and this is the premise of our work for It's Ok To Talk. Other expressions we hear commonly tend to frame mental health in a negative way (e.g., distress, sadness, difficulties, etc.) This insight is what has helped us re-frame our messaging more positively to amplify two simple key messages through Mann Mela — first, that everyone has mental troubles and, second, that mental health is one of our most positive assets.

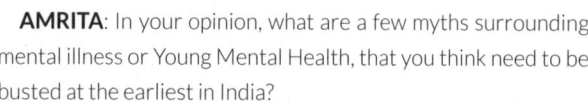

Young MENTAL HEALTH

AMRITA: In your opinion, what are a few myths surrounding mental illness or Young Mental Health, that you think need to be busted at the earliest in India?

PATTIE GONSALVES: Great question. These comprise of our programme's key messages! All myths turned around and derived from literature reviewing on mental health literacy and awareness amongst youth in India:

- That we ALL do not have mental health! — when in fact we are all human and all humans have mental health (mental health is our thoughts, feelings and behaviour and our ability to bounce back from the big and small stressors of life)
- That mental health is something to be feared — when in fact it is one of our biggest assets
- That everyone's mental health doesn't have ups and down
- That it's not OK to talk about our mental health
- That we cannot recover from a mental health problem

AMRITA: And finally, what would your message be to any adolescents/young adults reading this? And/or their families?

PATTIE GONSALVES: That it's not just OK — but vital — for us to be open and to talk about mental health.

Amrita Tripathi | Meera Haran Alva

DIAL ICALL FOR HELP: HOW THE TISS-HOUSED HELPLINE DELIVERS

Interview with iCall Helpline Programme Coordinator Tanuja Babre[39]

iCall is a psycho-social helpline run by the Tata Institute of Social Sciences (TISS), that aims to offer counselling via phone, mail and chat to those in emotional and psychological distress. The service which runs from 8 am to 10 pm from Monday to Saturday, is primarily funded by the Mariwala Health Initiative, since 2015.

The helpline has shared services to 80,000 clients (via call/ email and chat, etc.) till date and cites a follow-up rate of 64 per cent and — crucially — offers counselling services for free, in multiple languages: English, Hindi, Marathi, Tamil, Kannada, Gujarati, Bengali and Konkani. Stats apart, in a country that often doesn't seem to have enough affordable mental healthcare facilities or even resources to refer those in need to, iCall has long been a sort of silver lining.

The Health Collective's Sukanya Sharma interviewed iCall Programme Coordinator Tanuja Babre for more information and insight. Babre has a master's degree in counselling psychology from the Tata Institute of Social Sciences and has worked in the area of mental health and psychosocial well-being for over six years. Apart from offering services in a face to face setting, she has offered services for over 2,000 sessions via phone, email and chat.

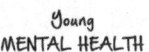
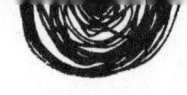

Young
MENTAL HEALTH

This interview first appeared on The Health Collective site around World Mental Health Day in 2019 and has been lightly edited for clarity.

1. WHAT WOULD YOU TELL PEOPLE WHO ARE FEELING SUICIDAL?

I think one of the crucial things to talk about in any kind of crisis prevention work is that there should be a message of hope that you should instil when talking to a user-survivor. When it comes to the issue of suicide, people often engage in these thoughts because they feel hopeless and worthless and probably don't see any other way to help them navigating through this particular situation. Therefore, any conversation that you are having, it is important that you are not being judgmental or taking a moralistic stance saying that , 'If you do this god will punish you', or 'If you do this, what will happen to your family?', or 'Think about your children', and so on.

It is important to create a safe space. It may so happen that you do not understand the reasons that they choose to do what they are doing but at the same time know that you are there to support them through this. It is also important to give a message of hope and communicate that you may not have the answers right now, but together (we) can figure out what the answers could be and (that) we will navigate through this. So, we need to be able to communicate that there is a way out of this, but also make sure that we do not make any false promises by saying, 'I'm going to resolve this for you'. Assuring (someone) that you and I will figure out how to get out of this situation, is the most important thing.

2. DO YOU HAVE A MESSAGE FOR FAMILY, FRIENDS, AND INSTITUTES ON HOW TO BE SENSITIVE?

One of the important things to remember is that there are a lot of myths around suicide and self-harm. One of the most common myths is that if you ask the person about this then you instil an idea about this in their mind. This is not true. If you see someone showing signs of being suicidal then it is important that you talk to them about whether they are thinking of ending their life, whether they are feeling vulnerable. You doing that is not going to put the idea in the person's head.

We have all witnessed experiences of suicide around us. Possibly we have all unfortunately lost loved ones through it, or friends or colleagues. Another point to note is that feeling suicidal may be a sign of depression, and it is not a way to get attention or manipulate someone.

If this is happening in an organisation, most commonly I've heard that the organisation sends the person on leave, saying that when they feel better, they should come back — that is not the healthiest thing to do, at that point of time. You need to ensure that you connect them to a mental health professional, a support system, someone from their family or any trusted adult who they are close to are informed about it so they can take care of them.

The new Mental Healthcare Act decriminalises suicide so I think there is a lot of education also that has to be done of the stakeholders around this particular change because healthcare professionals often fear liability and deny treatment in such cases.

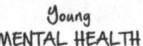

3. IS THERE A SPIKE IN THE NUMBER OF CALLS AROUND ANY PARTICULAR TIME OF THE YEAR?

Over the years that iCall has been functioning, we have noticed that during the exam season when the Board results are about to come out, is when we get a huge chunk of calls from students. Some of the students are worried about the outcome of the results, some call after the results are out and feel depressed. The concerns may be a little different for those who call after the results; they are more anxiety-related, saying: 'My parents are forcing me to take a certain career', 'Which institution to choose?', 'I have no plan B'…

4. HOW DOES A CALL FLOW?

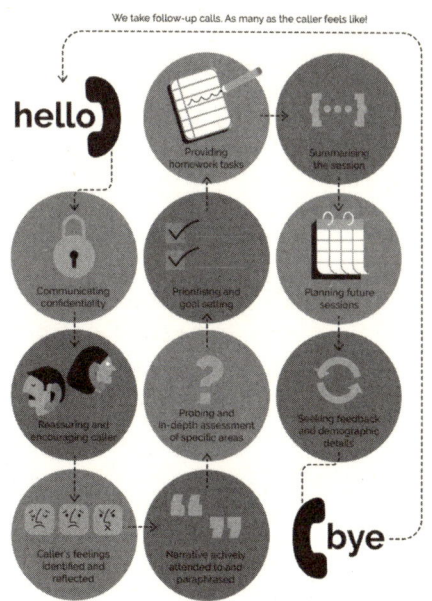

CALL PROTOCOL

Image courtesy: icallhelpline.org

5. HOW DOES THE CALL END?

This varies from case to cases. Depending on the issue the client has come to the counsellor with, the counsellor may provide short term intervention, sometimes they refer to an organisation that may be helpful or some reading material and they will set up an agenda for the next call. Sometimes counsellors also give the clients homework to do; coping cards, lists of things to engage in, and the client then has to come with that homework for the next session.

6. YOUNG SUICIDE RATES ARE A GROWING CONCERN — DO YOU GET MANY CALLS FROM THE YOUNGER DEMOGRAPHIC? WHAT ARE THEIR TRIGGERS? WHAT ARE SOME OF THEIR CONCERNS?

Almost 40 per cent of the people who get in touch with us are in the age group of 11–30 years. The topmost concerns that people are reaching out to us with are relationship concerns followed by sexuality related issues academic and career related, mental health related concerns, substance use, etc. These are some of the common concerns that young people are accessing our services with. The issue related to suicide is often attached to academics. We also used to run special service for students who are situated in the city of Kota. This is where the kids are going to train for their competitive exams for engineering and medicine. We got a lot of calls from clients who are feeling suicidal because of academic pressure, or experiencing violence/abuse happening through the coaching classes.

But there are also a lot of issues related to relationships; abuse, violence, breakup.

Some young people reach out with concerns of getting married or getting a divorce, there's violence in relationships. There are also clients who deal with difficulties with family members, being a care-giver to them, and feeling the care-giver fatigue.

7. ONE PER CENT OF THE CALLS COME IN FROM THE TRANSGENDER COMMUNITY. COULD YOU ELABORATE A LITTLE ON WHAT KIND OF CONCERNS THEY CALL YOU WITH? WHAT ARE SOME OF THE TRIGGERS?

Some of them may be related to transition. They are also at different levels of transition. Some say that they wish to do it: 'I identify like that but I don't know how to go about it.' 'Can you tell me what this is?' Some people call in to say that they feel different and that they need help to get rid of these feelings.

Some call in with their family members to help their families understand what this transition means and to sensitise them. Sometimes families reach out to say that they are okay with their loved ones living dual lives and they can do whatever in their private time. At times it is particularly challenging because some of them are married and they have partners and kids. Clients are also concerned how their families will react during this transition period.

There are also those who come with mental health concerns like depression. Some are stressed because of the discrimination they might be facing at the workplace, or in society and how they can get help around that. Some clients come with relationship issues with their partners — break-ups, or when both the partners transitioning, or if only one partner transitioning, separation, coming out to family members, etc.

8. WHAT KIND OF HELP DO COUNSELLORS GET?

Certainly, our work is taxing and complex. So there are certain mechanisms that we have evolved in the organisation over the years, and it's a constantly evolving process, to be honest.

- One of the few mechanisms in place is that every employee of iCall, whether a counsellor or admin staff or anyone, are given a therapy allowance on an annual basis whereby they can use the money to seek therapy for themselves. It can either be therapy or we have a list of activities that they can use that they think will help their mental health.
- We have supervision available for all counsellors. This operates at various levels: one is that they have access to peer supervision where their senior colleagues are available to them, there is also one-to-one supervision where a person is appointed to help the person through any issues.
- In the iCall office we even keep a lot of arts and crafts materials, there is food for the counsellors wherein they can put in their request for it. These are just some efforts to make the environment more friendly for them.

As an organisation, we like to believe that we are sensitive to people's needs and each of us is mindful of each other's mental health. The team will encourage frequent timeouts to make everyone feel less burdened ... each counsellor answers anywhere between 7-12 calls daily, and the duration of the call on an average is around 23 minutes.

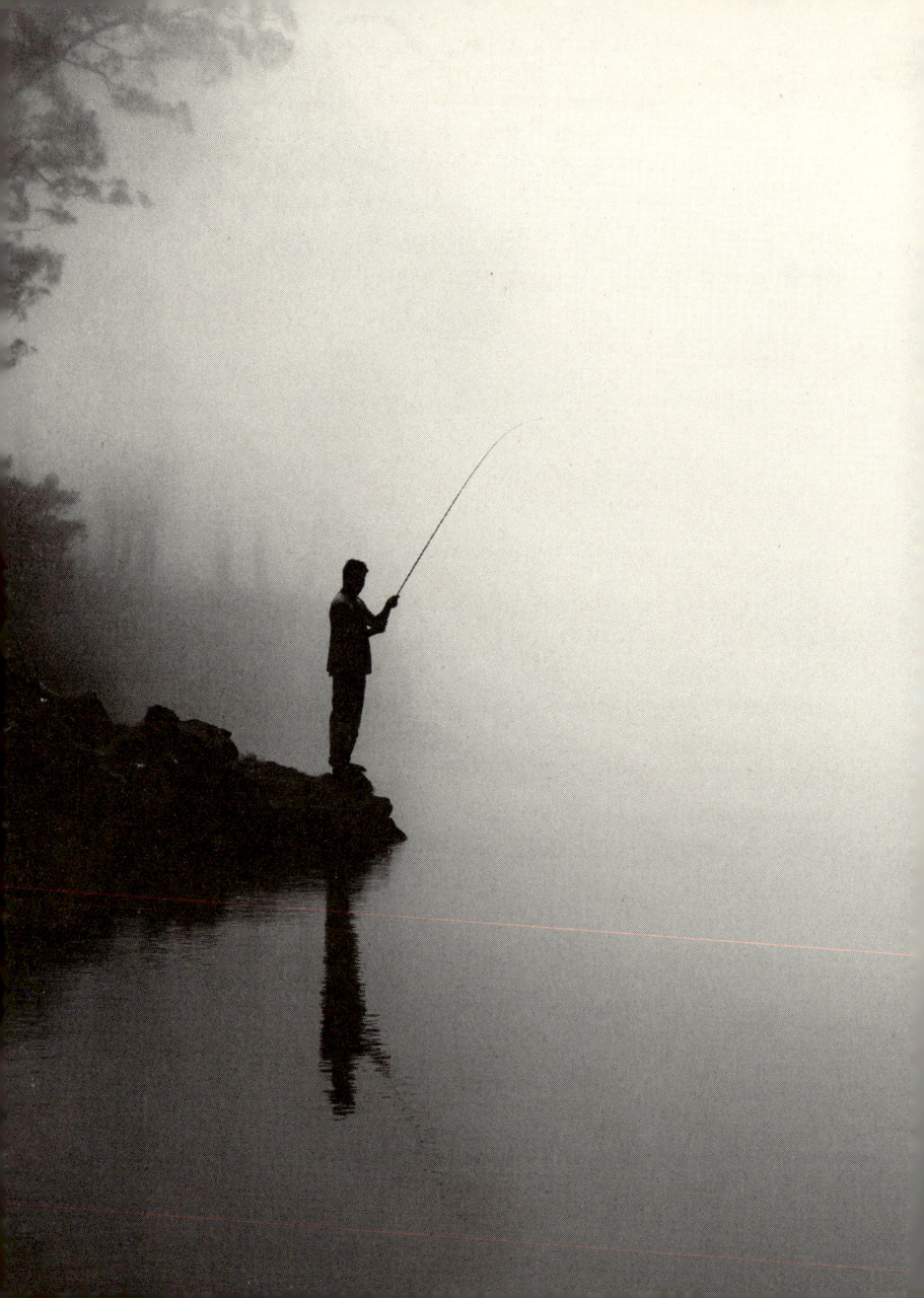

Chapter 13
IN THEIR OWN WORDS
Aftermath: Words and Art by Oz

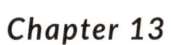

About the Artist: Oz describes his work as an aboriginal playground of all things scrap, a space of union for the freak derivatives of high and low cultures. He uses unconventional tones and dabbles in different media to paint his body of work, which surrounds themes of mythic, fantastic and bipolar natures. His works can be often found to bestow an ornate eye on the darker side of things. He believes there must somewhere be a place where all physical, virtual, and varied dimensional mediums can interact, and hence, is constantly gnawing for it. He also believes in anarchist aliens. Oz works as an illustrator and comic book artist, and sometimes finds himself moonlighting on different design consultations and commissions. He lives in Bangalore, India with friends and cats.

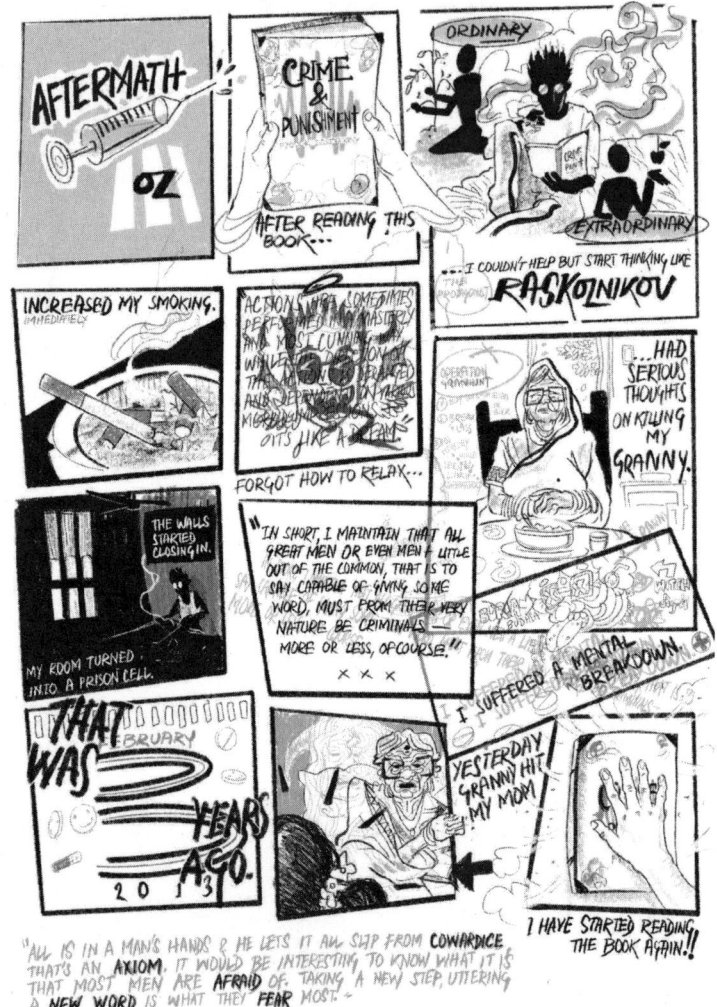

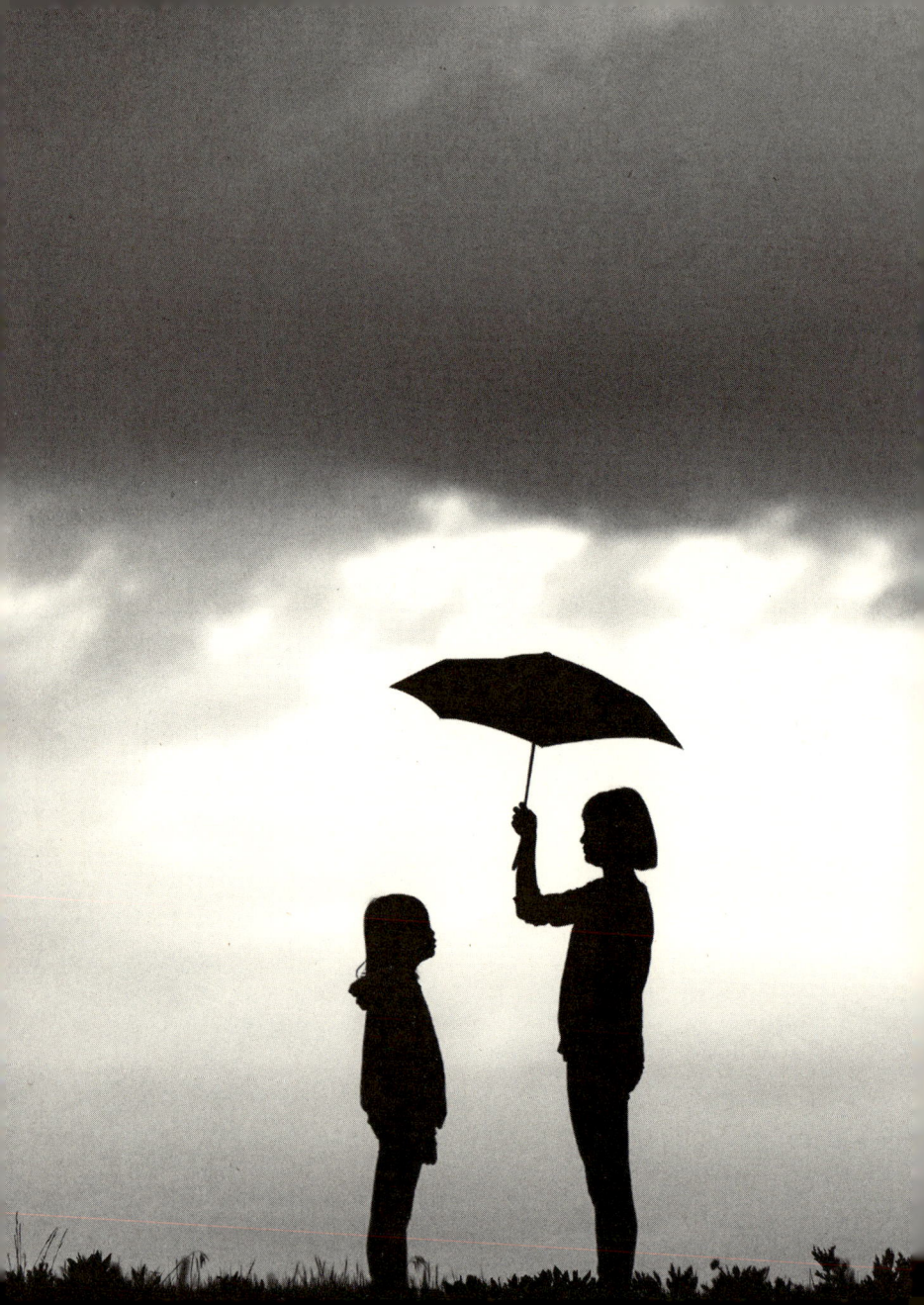

Chapter 14
FAQ'S AND A PRACTICAL HANDBOOK FOR PARENTS
By Meera Haran Alva

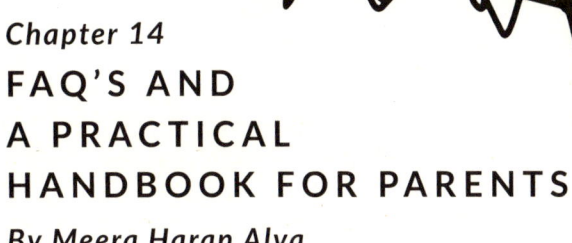

WHAT IS A NORMAL CHILD?
Parenting FAQ's and Understanding Therapy

'Is my child normal?' This is a question that I get asked frequently by many anxious parents. It is a question I can truly empathise with, as a mother myself.

As parents we unfortunately do not have a manual to guide us on how to handle the growing needs of our child at every stage — to know at times if how they are behaving is normal or if how we are responding to it is adequate. We rely on our instincts, learning from our own parent's mistakes or when they got it right with us and from extended family members who readily bail out advice whether we ask for it or not.

As our child grows, so do our concerns at different stages. I still remember the time when our son didn't walk even at 17 months; a developmental paediatrician told us that he had a gross motor delay of three months. This was very frightening for us to hear and we spent the next month getting him a walker and physiotherapy sessions. Our son did not budge at all and was happy crawling around exploring the world on his fours. And, one fine day he just got up and started walking. He is now a 10-year-old athletic child who is on the school football team, but who would have guessed that back then?! While I am relieved that my son didn't have a gross motor delay, I do realise that it was helpful that we followed our instincts and reached out for help when we noticed the delay and provided him with the necessary support and intervention. Unfortunately, what is often seen with emotional difficulties, mental health issues or disabilities of varying kinds is the delay in seeking help — a concern also shared by Dr Amit Sen in his earlier interview. The need for early intervention cannot be over-emphasised.

So, when does one seek professional help? To begin with, it is important to understand that each and every child is unique, different and wonderful in their own way. It is important to respect the fact that they learn, grow and develop at their own pace. Thus the debate of what is a part of normal development vs when does it become concerning becomes subjective especially when it comes to the need for intervention and therapy.

However, it is absolutely okay to seek therapy for 'normal' developmental stressors to help ease anxiety for the parent, normalise the difficulty and learn some strategies to help cope with it. In cases where you begin to experience or notice that there are difficulties that are affecting yours or your child's functioning on a regular basis (consistently) please do not hesitate or wait for it to escalate — seek support immediately.

From a psycho-education point of view, I would recommend learning about different developmental frameworks[40] that give you an outline of what you can expect at every stage of your child or adolescent's development and also help you understand their needs. These references can help normalise behaviours that seem 'appropriate' for the child's age and developmental stage. [41]

There are several developmental theories with respect to a child's or adolescent's physical, perceptual, cognitive, social and emotional development. References have been shared in the bibliography.

Due to the constraints of space I will be sharing a few developmental references for social and emotional development of adolescents. You could refer to these for your children in other age groups as well.

Erik Erikson, a prominent developmental psychologist of the 1950's developed the psychosocial theory of human development that covers the entire life span of the individual, including his adult life.[42] According to him, individual's progress through a series of stages as they grow and change throughout life. During each of these stages, the individual is faced with a developmental conflict that needs to be resolved successfully in order to develop the primary virtue of that stage. He was interested in how relationships and social interactions affect development and growth. Viewing adolescence from this perspective, Erikson explains the stage between the ages of 12-18 as the 'identity vs confusion' stage. During this stage, the conflict centers around the evolving sense of the individual's personal identity. Those who receive the needed encouragement and reinforcement through personal exploration tend to emerge from this phase with a strong sense of self and a feeling of independence and control. Those who remain unsure of their beliefs and desires will remain insecure and confused about themselves and the future.

Hence it is normative to see your adolescent behave in an unpredictable and impulsive way as this is the way that they can explore and find a sense of who they are. Parents want to continue exerting their influence on how their teens feel about themselves, but these may conflict with external forces such friends, social groups, societal trends, and even popular culture that may all play a significant role in shaping and forming the adolescent's identity.

Those who are not allowed to explore and test out different identities might be left with what Erikson referred to as role confusion. These individuals are not sure who they are or what they like. They tend to become socially disconnected and cut-off from others, they may drift from one job or relationship to another, never really sure what they want to do with their lives. Lacking this sense of who they are leaves them feeling disappointed and confused about their place in life.

Pamela Levine, a prominent transactional analyst who developed the 'cycles of development'[43], calls this stage of adolescent development the stage of 'integration'. She identifies the following developmental tasks for this stage:

- To take steps towards independence
- To achieve a clearer emotional separation from family
- To emerge as a separate independent person with own identity and values
- To be competent and responsible for own needs, feeling and behaviours
- To integrate sexuality into earlier developmental tasks

She also shares affirmations that the parent can give to the adolescent child for this stage. Affirmations are the messages parents can convey to encourage the child to attend to the tasks specific to the stage. This can be done verbally and or non-verbally via actions and communication.

Here are the affirmations for this stage:

- You can know who you are and learn and practice skills for independence
- You can develop your own interests, relationships and causes
- You can grow in your femaleness or maleness and still need help at times
- You can learn to use old skills in new ways
- We look forward to knowing you as an adult
- We trust you to ask for support when you need it

Failure to achieve this integration leaves the individual feeling somewhat fragmented, a sense of not having finished growing up. The part that I find to be most therapeutic about this model is that it is cyclic in nature and it gives us a chance to re-visit stages when we are unable to fulfil these tasks due to the lack of encouragement or affirmations from our parents or care-givers during our childhood and adolescence.

As an adult, how would you know if you might be revisiting this stage?

- When you find yourself exploring the same themes again, such as sex and its importance in our lives.
- When you find yourself exploring and revisiting your identity, values and personal philosophies.
- When you find yourself acting like a 'teenager', exploring music, drugs, experimenting sexually or having higher sleep needs.

In the Indian context[44], sex is a very sensitive subject and discussions on sexual matters are considered a taboo in Indian society. There is considerable stigma around having a conversation about sex with your children. While talking to

parents in sessions, what I gather is their own discomfort in talking about sexuality also includes their fear that discussing it would somehow indicate that they are endorsing it or being permissive about it.

The famous psychoanalyst Sigmund Freud's controversial psycho-sexual development theory[45] also emphasises the significance of adolescent sexuality. According to him, children go through a series of psychosexual stages that lead to the development of the adult personality.

Adolescence, according to this theory, is in the final stage of what he calls the 'Genital stage', which begins in puberty and lasts through the rest of the individual's life. It is a time of adolescent sexual experimentation, the successful resolution of which is settling down in a loving one-to-one relationship with another person in their adulthood. The greatest challenge of this stage is for the adolescent to have to balance their most basic urges against the need to conform to the demands of social and cultural norms.

As a parent, if you find it challenging to talk about puberty or sexuality with your adolescent, you could share resources with them that they can read when they are ready.[46] It would be helpful if you went through these resources yourself before you shared this information and then let them know that they can come back to you with questions.

If your own values and upbringing make it difficult for you to talk to your children about sexuality and relationships, you can discuss this with a school counsellor or a therapist off-campus. The professional can help you with any questions or concerns that you may have and can also have sessions with your adolescent if required.

A reminder: The need for help or support can be a good enough reason to seek therapy. It is valid and healthy to ask for help.

CASE ILLUSTRATION:
TEENAGER WITH IDENTITY AND SELF-WORTH ISSUE

(Through the lens of developmental frameworks)

*Names and all identifying details have been changed to protect the privacy of individuals

Lokesh* was a 16-year-old boy who was struggling with his identity and sense of self-worth. He referred himself to the therapist. When the therapist met him, he shared his struggles with his parents. They seemed to be very unhappy with him lately. They would get upset and easily distressed when he spent his time with his friends or locked up in his room listening to music. His parents even went to the extent of taking the locks off his door. They did not approve of his choice of music (punk metal) or his choice of clothing (torn jeans and 'loud' t- shirts).

They expected him to spend his time post-school with either the family or studying at his desk — all other activities according to them were a waste of his time. They urged him to take his academics seriously as the 12th Boards were coming up in a matter of a year's time. Lokesh was also dealing with peer-related conflicts at school. He was being bullied by a group of boys who made fun of his appearance as he was on the heavier side. He was unable to share this with his parents, as he was unsure of whether they would take it seriously or not.

REFLECTIONS:

• What we see here is Lokesh struggling with what seems like a normative part of adolescence. In the way that he is exploring his identity through music and clothing (referring to Erickson's identity vs role confusion). The therapist validated Lokesh's struggles and was interested in his explorations. In such cases it is helpful even when parents do not share the same interests as their children to actually make an effort to be curious about it and if they are daring, decide to learn more about it.

• Academic exam stress is often experienced as being equally stressful for both parents and their children. A negotiation of reasonable expectations from the parents of what the child can and cannot do is necessary in terms of planning their study time and routine. In this case the stress of the upcoming exams began to define the relationship between the parents and Lokesh — not leaving any scope for him to share anything else really, not even something as important and urgent as the issue of bullying that he was experiencing at school.

• Bullying needs to be taken seriously as Ananya Dhanuka points out in her powerfully written poetry on bullying in Chapter 10 of this book — 'everyone is a stakeholder'. I couldn't agree more. While we hope that Lokesh has the courage to stand up and speak for himself, we also acknowledge that the parents and teachers — systems that have the power to take action — actually do what is expected of them. The therapist encouraged Lokesh to report the bullying and the school did take action against the students who were bullying him. His parents were sad to hear that Lokesh did not have confidence in them to share his distress and were able to see the reasons why.

• The parents shared that they were finding it emotionally difficult to see Lokesh exert his independence and were trying to pull back. The therapist validated their anxiety and helped them understand their fears around this separation. As the therapist normalised this as being a part of Lokesh's adolescent development task to achieve a clearer emotional separation from his family (Reference Pamela Levine's cycle of development described earlier in this chapter), the parents began to ease up the control and work on the first affirmation of this stage: 'You can know who you are and learn and practice skills for independence'.

WHAT IS A FAMILY?

How we define 'the family' and 'what our family life should be like' is influenced by the ideologies and narratives in the context of the society or culture we live in at a given time in history.[47]

The challenge is that for many of us the image of the family that immediately comes to mind is of a nuclear family unit of a husband and wife with children born to them. Any other forms of family are seen as a deviation from this norm and are judged as 'not normal'. Single parenthood, an unmarried couple living together, a gay couple adopting a child, divorced couple parenting their children together are examples of 'other forms of family' that are seen as being far from the ideal.

There needs to be a change of interpretation in how we view the evolving forms of family life. To see this as an evolution of family practices that have developed over time in response to culture, history, socio-economic practices, gender relationships rather than a breakdown of society. [48]

FAMILY LIFE CYCLE

The family life cycle can be seen as a series of stages with a set of tasks that family members need to complete in order to go to the next. When there are difficulties in completing these tasks, families may then experience adjustment problems.[49] Families follow common patterns as they change and develop through the different life cycle stages. These changes are shaped by the internal and external demands of society. [50]

Internal pressures to change:

- Biological: Growth, change and development
- Social/psychological needs, expectations, roles, etc.
- Family organisation: Rules, hierarchy, intimacy, alliances

External pressures to change:

- School
- Friends
- Leisure
- Cultural expectations
- Extended family
- Work

The internal and external changes are continuous but become critical at transitional points in family life. These variations in life cycle stages differ culturally as do the ideas around belief systems, forms of family, types of marriages, parent–child relationships and extended family relationships.

Families need to make changes at these critical transitional points, such as changing the family structure, beliefs or emotional dynamics. It has been seen that emergence of problems are frequently associated with these life cycle transitions that bring with it inherent demands and stresses. These developmental stressors are normative, however, they may manifest in different ways in families.

FAMILIES WITH YOUNG CHILDREN

During this stage parents may face difficulties with children that often arise from the struggles they may be experiencing with the generation gap between them and their children. For instance, they may find their children 'impossible to control' or 'too playful', expecting children to behave more like adults.

One of the main challenges in this phase is of sharing childcare responsibilities and household chores. With changes in employment practices and issues of gender roles changing, in more families we see that both parents have full time jobs and the adverse consequences are experienced by the family: responsibilities of both jobs often falls on the woman, the family is on a tight budget to accommodate child care services, there may be neglect or abuse of the child whilst in child care or the woman may end up giving up her job to stay at home or do part time work to care for the child. At the core, these issues may lead to marital conflict.[51]

FAMILIES WITH ADOLESCENTS

Families experience transformation during adolescence and there are certain universal problems associated with this transition.

One of the main challenges of this phase is of parents coming to terms with how they no longer maintain complete authority as they did when their children were younger. The time comes for them to re-negotiate and work towards establishing qualitatively different boundaries with their adolescent allowing them to develop autonomy. This is an extremely complex and demanding stage especially for parents.

Cultural contexts play an important role in how different families negotiate the rules and limits, which are key during this stage of development. In urban India, our cultural values are evolving as we find our family systems changing. Shagufa Kapadia did an interesting study on adolescent-parent relationships in the Indian context, where she studied the nature of everyday disagreements that occur between parents and adolescents across two very distinct cultures i.e. Indian and American.[52] She studied how these disagreements were resolved, to what extent were the adolescents able to consider their parent's perspective whilst making sense and resolving these disagreements and also to compare the perspective differences between Indian adolescents and Indian immigrant adolescents (in the US).

The results indicated that adolescents cross culturally experienced everyday disagreements related to:
- Regulation of behaviour or activities
- Interpersonal relationships
- Academics
- Chores
- Finance

The strategies commonly used across these contexts to resolve these disagreements were:

- Compromise on behalf of the adolescent and
- Mutual accommodation

It is interesting to note that a larger number of Indian adolescents acknowledged their responsibility to accommodate their parent's views. This was on account of their faith in the parents' experiences, their respect for them and the belief that parents have their children's welfare at heart. Adolescents from both the groups also endorsed the need for parent accommodation to adolescent views while the need for parent compromise featured more in the Indian immigrant group.

I see this in my clinical practice as I find myself having to advocate for the adolescent's need for independence while respecting the need for the parent's responsibility and concern to protect their adolescent.

In her chapter 'Transformation of Family System during Adolescence', Nydia Garcia Preto shares key areas of challenges faced by families with adolescents and suggests what families can do to address these issues[53]:

• RENEGOTIATING RELATIONSHIPS BETWEEN PARENTS AND ADOLESCENTS: As parents and their adolescent children renegotiate their relationship during adolescence, parents often experience a resurfacing of unresolved issues with regard to their own parents. It is helpful for parents to think about their own childhood and adolescence and reflect on their own relationships with their parents — this understanding could be very helpful in furthering their ability as a parent to listen and feel less reactive to their children's behaviour.

• BUILDING A COMMUNITY: Culturally, we are in transition now, moving away from traditional joint family systems to living in a nuclear family system.. We need to make an effort to reach out to others, as it can be very challenging to raise adolescents without any support.

Parents need support and encouragement to:

- Hang in there
- Listen differently
- Confront their own limits
- Take necessary measures to earn their children's trust

Parents can do this by making connections and sharing their difficulties with other parents, empathetic extended family members, friends and professionals.

• STRENGTHENING THE PARENTAL BOND: It is quite common to see parents focusing on their adolescent's issues at the cost of neglecting their own couple relationship. Whether parents are together or separated, they need to agree on the rules for their children. The adolescent can often be seen triangulated between their parent's struggles. Alliances formed between one of the parents with the child further escalates the stress. The case of 16-year-old Lakshmi illustrates her difficulties as she is in a triangle between her parents who are in conflict.

CASE ILLUSTRATION: THE PARENT-CHILD BOND*

* Names and all identifying details have been changed to protect the privacy of individuals

Lakshmi's parents had dreams of her becoming a medical doctor but as Lakshmi entered her high school years she had become interested in dance and wanted to pursue a career in the performing arts. Her parents disapproved of her choices and this led to arguments and high stress levels at home. Lakshmi began to withdraw from her peers and started missing a lot of school. This change in her behaviour concerned both her teachers and parents. They referred her to a therapist. During the sessions, it became clear that Lakshmi was caught in a classic triangle of trying to please her parents and feeling responsible for their arguments. What also surfaced was the deep dissatisfaction that the parents had felt in their marriage and focusing their attention and energy on Lakshmi and this dream of seeing her become a doctor brought meaning and reason for them to stay on in this relationship.

REFLECTIONS:

- The therapist helped the parents take a step back from planning Lakshmi's future and let her take responsibility for her career choices. They were encouraged to be curious about her interest in the performing arts and work toward understanding her expectations from what she wanted to do in college. This helped strengthen their bond with Lakshmi.
- The parents also worked on their own adolescent and family of origin issues. This helped them become clearer about differentiating between the past and present.
- They also focused on their relationship issues and paid attention to working on their marriage thus freeing Lakshmi to pursue dreams that were her own.

UNDERSTANDING THERAPY: WHAT IS FAMILY THERAPY?

The interdisciplinary study of how different systems influence the individual and maintain difficulties underpins family therapy. In this form of therapy the emphasis is upon working with different members of a family or system. This is what sets family therapy apart from other psychotherapy approaches that focus on the individual.

There are many theories in family therapy, some focus on the role of the family in predisposing certain members to developing the problems for instance if a child is refusing to go to school — the child is not seen as the problem but the family dynamics are explored to understand why the child feels he needs to stay at home.

In such a case, it could be that the parents are going through conflict and the child feels the need to stay at home and support his mother.

Other theories focus on the role of the family in problem maintenance. For example, if a teenager is getting into trouble with late night partying, drinking and doing drugs — the focus is not on the teenager being the problem to fix, it is about how the family is responding to this problem. The parents may not have clear boundaries or limits set for her. She may have access to money to maintain her lifestyle. There may not be clear communication between the family members on what is accepted and appropriate behaviour. Thus the family plays a role in maintaining this problem and the therapist focuses on working with them to establish clearer boundaries and better communication between members of the family.

Still, other theorists have broadened family therapy to include members of the wider professional and social networks around the family. This is called 'systemic practice'. An example for this would be if a child were being bullied at school, the family therapist would work with the school and family to ensure that both systems are aware and in sync with regards to ensuring that the child feels safe. While the school implements their discipline policy with regards to bullying and works with children who are bullying the concerned child, the therapist also works with the child and family to alleviate the anxiety and provide them with support and effective strategies to cope with the situation. There are times when the therapist sits with the family and school to help them have conversations about the child's concerns. The therapist mediates these conversations and also advocates for the child's well-being.

'THE SECURE CHILD': FROM A SYSTEMIC PERSPECTIVE

When understanding children, it is helpful to recognise that the two most influential systems in their development are the family and school. To explain this further, it would help to understand the Attachment Theory of the psychologist John Bowlby, who revolutionised the field of child development.

According to Bowlby, who developed the Attachment Theory, children who had secure attachments with their parents were able to explore the world knowing that their parents are available when they were anxious or distressed. This secure attachment provides them with the safety to be free and autonomous. On the other hand, insecure children are more likely to have emotional issues by the time they are ready for school and have difficulties with attention and peer relationships.

Parents are able to have secure attachments with their children when they have a clear understanding of their children's needs and vulnerabilities. Parents who are unable to empathise with their children tend to have insecure relationships.

This theory of parent-child attachments has been extended to the understanding of how the family can provide a secure base from which children can explore and develop.[54] Now, within the family system, if the parents and other significant members are not supportive of each other and they involve the child as an alliance in their battle with the other parent, this can affect the security of the child, where she experiences divided loyalties and loses out on appropriate parental care. In such cases whether or not the parents are separated, the child ends up becoming a partner rather than the child of that parent.

When parents begin working on their own conflicts, children begin to feel freer, secure and are able to attend to their own lives.

Similar to how family attachments influence security, is recognising that the two key social systems in the child's life: the school and family being supportive of each other makes a child feel more secure. On the contrary, if a child who is experiencing difficulties senses that there is mistrust between these systems they feels insecure and experiences emotional distress. Collaboration between all adults is a significant factor for a child's well-being. [55]

FAMILY THERAPY FOR CHILDREN AND ADOLESCENTS

There is evidence-based research indicating that family therapy is effective for a range of disorders in children and adolescents. It has been found to be a useful therapeutic approach for:

- Mood and eating disorders
- Anxiety disorders
- Sleep, feeding and attachment problems in infancy
- Recovery from child abuse and neglect
- Conduct problems, emotional problems, eating disorders and somatic problems[56]

CASE ILLUSTRATION: THE FAMILY THERAPY PROCESS*

*Names and all identifying details have been changed to protect the privacy of individuals

Neelam came to see a family therapist, as she was concerned about her 13-year-old daughter, Sapna. Sapna had been very anxious lately and was having sleep difficulties. The lack of sleep had thrown her completely off balance and she was unable to attend to her school-work and was lagging behind in class, which further triggered her anxiety.

During the first meeting, the family therapist learnt that Neelam was a single mother since Sapna's birth. She and her father had separated when Sapna was only a few months old. There had been no contact with the father ever since. The mother and daughter had moved to three different cities as work for Neelam involved job transfers. During the sessions Sapna had revealed that her mother had been hiding a secret from her. She had overheard Neelam talking to a man in a tone that suggested that he might be her boyfriend. Sapna continued to 'investigate' and found more evidence to support her hunch.

Neelam acknowledged that this was true and that she had met Ramesh at her workplace and had recently begun dating him. In their small family unit this was the first time that Neelam was in a relationship since the divorce and she was fearful of sharing this information with her daughter, as she was unsure of how her daughter would respond to this. She too was anxious about the impact this would have on their close bond.

In subsequent sessions, Sapna also shared her anxiety of losing her mother to Ramesh and that everything would change and she did not want that to happen. She also felt betrayed that her mother, Neelam, had not disclosed this information to her earlier on. As the therapy continued and the hidden fears of both mother and daughter came into the open, Neelam was able to offer Sapna support and assurance. They talked about the challenges and stress they had faced individually and as a family through their many moves. Sapna had talked about her anger towards her mother for 'making her move cities' and for all the friends she had lost in the process. Neelam acknowledged this and empathised with her daughter's experiences. This sharing and listening helped strengthen and heal their relationship.

The two-member family decided that it would be helpful for Sapna to also have individual sessions with the therapist to talk about her school-related issues due to their many moves. Sapna began to feel better through the course of these sessions and her anxiety symptoms improved.

The family re-visited the therapist a year later when Neelam decided to tie the knot with Ramesh. The three of them began attending sessions together to work on their 'new family unit'.

This case illustrates:

- A different form of family, where the mother is a single parent and the head of the household.
- The initial referral was with the mother identifying her child as having sleeping difficulties. Instead of focusing on the child as being the 'problem', the family therapist focuses on the mother–daughter relationship. Together, they work through the secrets and fears that the family experienced as a result of the possible changes in their family unit. This illustrates how families often bring children to therapy as the 'symptom' bearer of a much deeper issue located in the family dynamics that then gets revealed through the therapy process.
- One of the big stressors for this family is of them feeling anxious about an upcoming change in their family life cycle, Neelam's 're-marriage' to Ramesh. Neelam's courtship with Ramesh brings changes in the family composition. This life cycle transition brings with it demands for change and adaptation from the family unit of the mother and daughter.

TOOL BOX FOR FAMILIES

There are creative, therapeutic tools used by family therapists to help engage families in therapy. This helps ease therapy from an adult treatment approach (verbal) to include an attitude of 'play' for all the members. It has been found that play is the language of children and when families can see the value of communicating with their children in this way, often symbolically, significant improvements are possible. [57]

I would like to share a few of these tools that you could use at home with your families to have more engaging conversations especially involving children and adolescents. It is important to be mindful that you make it safe for all members of the family especially the children to express their point of view or representation of how they see things without any responses from the others that are critical, threatening, minimising or dismissive. Family members can use this as a space to be curious about each other in a respectful way. These tools can help members express their thoughts, feelings and concerns leading to a stronger connection between family members. Instances when the issues or difficulties at hand seem way too challenging or overwhelming, do not hesitate to reach out for professional support.

TOOL#1 – FAMILY DRAWINGS:

Each of the members of the family draws their idea of how they see their family on a sheet of paper. You can then talk about what you have drawn in turns and ask each other questions about the other's drawings. In my reflections with the family, I have found that the family begins to ask each other lots of questions and interesting revelations are made — how come is it that you haven't drawn your father in the picture? ('because he is never around'); who is this person next to you mother? ('it's Thathi [grandmother], even though she is dead Amma misses her a lot').

It is surprising to see how and who each of the family members add to this picture. It is not just the drawing but also the explanations that go along with them that can be very revealing. I must share that pets are an all-time favourite addition to family drawings. In Indian families, you can often see that nannies, grandparents, uncles/aunts and nieces are included in the family drawing. This is because Indian families have a very different family organisation compared to the West due to their differing world-views and ideas of self.[58]

I once had a teenager who drew me in his family drawing; the child explained he couldn't imagine his family being together in the same room if it were not for the therapy space I offered. I was symbolic of the role of therapy in their lives. This was a powerful metaphor to understand what this child believed was holding his family together.

You could also add timelines to these drawings — asking each other to draw the family in the past, present and future or around significant milestones or life events. It could be with respect to significant changes in the family — divorce or deaths or a big move. Once I had a child draw her family looking rather happy in the past and this was when she was the only child — the first born. In the subsequent drawings there was a noticeable look of gloom and sadness in the drawings explaining how she felt with the loss of the attention and her place in the family.

TOOL#2 – CREATE YOUR FAMILY TREE:

This is another really helpful tool used in psychotherapy. I have found it effective when I work with individuals, especially adolescents and young adults. It's also a great way to engage the family to learn about family history and trans-generational information. This could be done on a large poster where you could draw a 'genogram' together. There are good references online on how to make a genogram.

Alternatively, there are also many free online 'family tree creator' websites and apps. This tool is suitable for all forms of families. For instance, those that are intact, single parent, LGBTQ, divorced families; families that have experienced a death, sexual abuse or depression. You can reveal relational dynamics between individuals while connecting them in the family tree. It may also reveal family secrets and alliances.

TOOL#3 – CREATE A FAMILY COLLAGE:

Family members make a collage together of pictures and words that they cut out from magazines or newspapers that describe how they feel about their family life. They can randomly glue their pictures or choices of words on a poster board. Members can discuss the reason for their choices and encourage each other to explain their perceptions about their family life, supporting their enjoyment of the positives and exploring solutions when problem areas are presented.

HOW DOES CHILD AND ADOLESCENT THERAPY WORK?

Child and adolescent therapy is a type of psychotherapy that refers to a variety of techniques and methods used to help children and adolescents who are experiencing difficulties with their emotions or behaviour.

INITIAL SESSIONS: ASSESSMENT

As part of the initial assessment, qualified mental health professional such as a psychotherapist or child and adolescent psychiatrist will determine the need for psychotherapy.

The initial session(s) is with the parent where the mental health professional will assess what support the child/ parent/family is looking for. The psychotherapist will then ask questions such as why is help being sought now? Who is most concerned/ worried about the child?

What do the school/ teachers or any other significant members of the family feel with regard to what the mental health professionals call the 'presenting' issue?

This assessment process may involve more than one session and the therapist will ask the parent about their child's or adolescent's history and may talk to other members of the family and school to understand the course of therapy. Research has shown that eating disorders, behavioural issues or school refusals are often a symptom of family or marital conflict and in such a case, family therapy seems most effective. This session thus is also a time to determine what form of therapy would best suit the family and meet their needs for support.

CONSENT

The consent of both parents is required when working with the child individually.

This can be a challenge when the parents are separated and one of them is not open to giving consent. In such cases the therapist would invite the non-consenting parent for an individual session to understand his/her concerns for their unwillingness for therapy and help them see the benefits for their child.

CONFIDENTIALITY

Confidentiality is at the core of therapy. Mental health professionals are required to state the confidentiality clause in the first session and maintain it through therapy. The confidentiality agreement is that the information shared by the child/adolescent with the therapist is strictly confidential except when the child/adolescent communicates threat to self or to another or if there is reasonable suspicion of child abuse — the information would then be disclosed to parents or other family members or the legal authorities.

This confidentiality agreement can be shared verbally or in a written signed document. This holds true in any setting where therapy takes place.

FREQUENCY AND LENGTH OF THERAPY SESSIONS

Typically, psychotherapy sessions are weekly. The frequency is determined based on the need and severity of the issue. In severe cases of anxiety or depression or other mental health issues, the therapist may even see a child on a thrice-a-week basis and taper it down over the course of therapy as things begin to improve.

The length of psychotherapy depends on the complexity and severity of problems and orientation of the therapist. Therapists who follow the solution-focused brief therapy methods, as the name suggests, work for a brief number of sessions, this can also be the case for cognitive behaviour therapists. For systemic therapists the termination or conclusion of therapy is a collaborative decision made by the therapist and client together. School-based counselling sessions are usually short term due to the context and nature of the services that can be time bound.

Psychotherapists of the humanistic-existential, person-centred and psycho-dynamic approaches follow a more long-term view of therapy and the end of therapy is usually determined by the client.

FORMS OF CHILD AND ADOLESCENT THERAPY

The professional in her initial sessions assesses and then recommends whether the child would benefit from

- Individual therapy
- Parent sessions
- Family and systemic therapy
- Group therapy
- Multi-family therapy
- School-based counselling

INDIVIDUAL THERAPY WITH CHILDREN

In individual therapy, a therapist provides a safe space for a child to be able to express himself through playing, drawing, building and pretending, as well as talking. Play is the most organic way in which a child interacts and expresses herself. Through the various forms of play, the therapist is then able to access the unconscious and unexpressed parts of the child's inner world that are difficult for the child to verbalise.

PARENT SESSIONS

A quote I read that really resonated with me and might have the same impact on parents reading this is by Karl Menninger, who is quoted[59] as saying, 'Being a parent, whether father or mother, is the most difficult task humans have to perform. For people, unlike other animals, are not born knowing how to be parents. Most of us struggle through.'

Parent support sessions can help address the concerns that parents may have with regard to their children's mental health. This decision of whether your child needs therapy can be made in your initial assessment session with the therapist.

Parent sessions can go hand in hand and run parallely along with the individual therapy sessions that take place with children or adolescents. Parent can benefit from support during the difficult and challenging transitions and developmental stages of their children. This stress is developmentally normative and yet it can have varied impacts on the individual parent based on their own personal life history and narrative. Seeking support for yourself as a parent can help you support your child more effectively and help raise them with more resolve.

Young
MENTAL HEALTH

The parent's mental health is a crucial determinant to the child's mental health and well-being. We have seen this with every development phase right from conception. For instance, perinatal depression is associated with increased risk for a child's emotional problems that can persist into young adulthood. Early identification and treatment of perinatal depression are critical to ensure optimal infant development and the child's future mental health.[60]

There have been many instances when parent support in therapy alone has helped alleviate the problem. During parent support sessions the therapist empathises with the parent, offers them psycho-education with regard to what their child may be experiencing developmentally and offers some strategies to deal with the stress associated with this time in their lives. The feeling of validation and support from the therapist and strategies to cope, in itself can help the parent feel more equipped to help support their child.

CASE ILLUSTRATION: PARENT SUPPORT*

*Names and all identifying details have been changed to protect the privacy of individuals

Bakul, a young mother, was concerned that her six-year-old daughter Aisha was unable to separate from her and attend 'big' school in the 1st standard. She contacted the school counsellor for support. In the sessions she shared that Aisha would be tearful and would throw the biggest tantrums when it was time to leave for school.

REFLECTIONS:

• The therapist assured Bakul that the first time a child leaves home for formal schooling it marks a significant developmental milestone in the family's life and can be anxiety provoking for both the parent and the child.

- The therapist validated Bakul's anxiety and normalised her feelings.
- She also invited the father Amir to join the parent support sessions. The idea behind this was for Amir to step in and share the responsibility of helping Aisha with this separation.
- And as Amir became more involved in the morning 'leaving for school' routines the pressure on Bakul to do this alone decreased and the goodbyes became less painful and the child was able to leave for school in a more secure way within a week.

FAMILY AND SYSTEMIC THERAPY

Please see the previous section for more detail on family and systemic therapy. I do want to point out that the field of family therapy is developing at a steady pace in urban India. There is a growing interest in working with families from a systemic family therapy perspective, but there are some infrastructural challenges. There are still no full-fledged training programmes in family therapy in India except for short-term courses offered by NIMHANS, and TISS.

In my clinical experience I still see fewer families than individuals in therapy. In practice, I find there is still apprehension for family members to seek therapy. Invariably, I end up seeing a family member or two but it is most challenging to get all members of a family to participate. The systemic approach, however, can be helpful when we work with individuals, especially with children. We ask questions about other family members in ways that brings them into the session without them even having to show up for therapy. This lends us understanding of what might be happening from a relational perspective in the family context.

From a child and adolescent therapy perspective, working with the family and the school of the child makes therapy more effective. Collaborating between the significant adults and systems in a child's life helps the child feel more secure and supported.

CASE ILLUSTRATION: INDIVIDUAL, FAMILY AND SYSTEMIC THERAPY*

*Names and all identifying details have been changed to protect the privacy of individuals

Rahul, a parent, contacted the therapist as he was worried about his eight-year-old son, Zubin, who was not talking in school. The class teachers had spoken to him about how Zubin was non- communicative in all class activities, including his interactions in the play area. The parents, Rahul and Archana, were surprised to hear this as Zubin was quite expressive and verbal at home.

REFLECTIONS:

- The therapist referred Zubin to a child and adolescent psychiatrist who diagnosed him with selective mutism, a social anxiety disorder where the child is capable of speech but cannot speak in specific situations or to specific people.
- The therapist worked from a systemic perspective, wherein she saw Rahul and Archana in parent support sessions, Zubin in individual play therapy sessions and his teachers to help support Zubin in school.
- As a result of the session with the teachers, they developed an I.E.P. — an individualised educational plan that included teacher education, accommodations and interventions for Zubin.
- The therapist found Zubin responded well to play therapy. He played by creating mini-worlds that were made up of miniature figures — showing the therapist glimpses of his inner world. There were dragons and armed men surrounding homes with little children. A lot of his depictions were that of fear and impending

danger. As the sessions progressed, he was able to express himself through play and a few scattered words. Through the course of therapy there was an improvement in the symptoms and he began very slowly engaging in communication, even if it were minimal, in the classroom settings.

- Unfortunately, the therapist could not continue her work with the family, as they had to move to another country unexpectedly due to the parent's job transfer.

This is an example to show systemic work — where we work in therapy with the child, family and the school system. This is also a case that indicates how play lends a safe space for children to express themselves and resolve their difficulties.

GROUP THERAPY

In some cases, therapists refer children and adolescents for group therapy, though this is still uncommon in India, it is slowly on the rise. Group therapy is commonly seen for addiction therapy — the Al-Anon and Alateen (a peer support group for teens) groups organise group therapy sessions in different parts of India for children, teens and families suffering both directly and indirectly the consequences of alcoholism and other addictions. For more information you can check online for their websites.

MULTI-FAMILY THERAPY

Another type of therapy work, again uncommon in India, but proving to be effective in the West for particular mental health issues is the multi-family therapy work. This is when the therapist works with multiple families and the focus is on enhancing the families' own adaptive mechanism and mobilising family strengths as a treatment approach. I have had the privilege of working with Dr. Ivan Eisler[61] as a family therapy trainee in his multi-family therapy research programme that has shown to be a promising treatment for adolescent anorexia nervosa.

SCHOOL-BASED COUNSELLING

In most school settings in India, school counsellors are not clinically trained. Therefore it is important to ascertain the qualifications of the counsellor depending on your referral concerns, before choosing them to work with your child. Like other mental health professionals, school counsellors use the initial meeting to assess whether they are able provide the support needed or if the child and family would benefit from a referral off campus.

A school counsellor could be considered when your concerns are school-related issues, such as helping new students adjust in school, peer-related issues, bullying issues, teacher-related problems, etc. These are situations where a school counsellor is able to liaison with other members of the school community in an effort to provide support for the child and parents.

For more serious issues such as anxiety or depression, eating disorders, abuse, etc., the child and family would benefit from seeking therapy off-campus from a professional who is qualified to work with these issues.

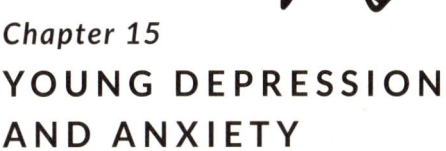

Chapter 15
YOUNG DEPRESSION AND ANXIETY

As you will have gathered, there are many implications of Mental Health issues, some of which can be life-long, which is why we feel that early identification and intervention are so important. I do sometimes have people asking me, 'Why are we identifying so many more disorders now?' or even, 'I never got diagnosed when I was young, and look I turned out okay', and my response to this is that it's not an 'all or nothing conversation' — our attempts to create awareness is not with the purpose to diagnose everyone but at the same time we cannot live in denial of existing mental health issues. It is helpful to re-frame this narrative, acknowledging the concern that lies at the heart of some of these statements and misconceptions.

It is extremely important for parents and even teachers to know how to have conversations about these issues, without minimising or dismissing them as trivial. We want to ensure children get the attention and help they might need early on, which can include support or intervention that helps address certain concerns that do not then lead to more serious challenges in their adult life.

The goal of this chapter is to help raise awareness about anxiety and depression in children and adolescents, and equip you with the tools you need, to have conversations about these pertinent issues without being in a rush to label others. A diagnosis needs to serve you and empower you- not the other way around.

We owe it to our younger generations to be more aware — and in my opinion, it is that awareness which is helping us notice and identify those who need help and support the most. I want to share some of the questions that often come up, which trouble parents. But keep in mind that these are indicative, and as I've mentioned before, not to be used for self-diagnosis!

ARE MOOD SWINGS A SIGN OF DEPRESSION?

Less than three decades ago, depression was seen as a predominantly adult disorder: children were considered developmentally immature to experience depressive disorders, and adolescent low mood was seen as part of 'normal' teenage mood swings. Developmental studies have been central in modifying that view. Few would now doubt the reality of child and adolescent depressive disorders, or that youth depression is associated with a range of adverse outcomes including social and educational impairments as well as both physical and mental health problems later in life.[62]

Depression is a mental health illness that affects how you feel, the way you think and how you act. Behaviour in children varies from one development stage to another. The challenge parents often face is to be able to differentiate in their child's behaviour and understand whether it is just a phase that their child is going through or if there is a reason for concern.

It must be noted that only a medical practitioner can diagnose a mental health illness such as depression. Psychiatrists follow a manual called the DSM ie 'Diagnostical Statistical Manual of Mental Disorders' or the 'International Classification of Diseases (ICD) . These manuals offer a common language and standard criteria for the classification of mental disorders. The DSM and ICD manuals are revised periodically to make it more relevant and current with research. The DSM-5 and ICD-11 are the latest revisions of these manuals. For the purpose of the writing of this book, I have referred to the DSM-5.

WHAT TO LOOK OUT FOR?

Please be cautioned not to self-diagnose your children's mental health. Always remember to consult a qualified mental health professional for a diagnosis. The DSM-5 is a manual that outlines specific criteria to help professionals diagnose mental health illnesses. Using DSM-5 as a reference[63], here is what you need to look out for as signs of depression:

If your child experiences five or more of the symptoms listed below most of the day, nearly every day for at least a two week period:

- Is your child in a depressed mood?
- Does s/he have diminished interest or pleasure in most activities?
- Have you noticed significant weight loss when not dieting or weight gain, or decrease or increase in appetite?
- Is there a slowing down of thought and a reduction of physical movement?
- Do you find your child fatigued or experiencing a loss of energy?
- Is she feeling worthless, hopeless about her future, or guilty about things that aren't her fault?

- Does s/he seem to have diminished ability to think or concentrate or seems indecisive?
- Does s/he have recurrent thoughts of death, recurrent suicidal ideation without a specific plan, or a suicide attempt or a specific plan for committing suicide? If so it's crucial you have your child evaluated by a mental health professional immediately. If the thoughts are really serious and there is imminent threat, you will need to take your child to the emergency department at the nearest hospital. (For some all-India helpline numbers, please refer to the Introduction of this book.)

To receive a diagnosis of depression, these symptoms shared above must cause the child significant distress or difficulties in important areas of functioning such as learning in school/college or socialising with peers, etc. The symptoms must also not be a result of substance abuse or any another medical condition.

If you suspect that your child has depression, talk to them and check with them on how they are feeling. Children may respond that they are sad or unhappy while others will say that they want to hurt themselves or to die. These statements should be taken very seriously. Please escalate any concerns to a trained mental health expert. You will find various lists of professionals and helplines collated, including at the end of this book. You can also check for word-of-mouth references. Please do not attempt to use this book or any information here to make a self-diagnosis or to diagnose anyone yourself.

I have noticed that children almost always confide in someone about their self-harming acts and somehow no one takes them seriously and hence they hesitate to share this with anyone. Sadly, self-harming behaviour is dismissed as attention-seeking behaviour and children are often shamed when their parents find out about it. Self-harming behaviour is a cry for help and needs to be attended to with urgency.

Escalate any such behaviour to the concerned experts.

DIFFERENTIATING BETWEEN SADNESS AND DEPRESSION

What do you think is the difference between feeling sad and depressed? Do you use these terms interchangeably? What do you feel is the difference?

During my sessions with children and adolescents, I find that for most of my young clients, the feeling of sadness is transient — it would stay for a short time and it was usually felt in response to an external event. For instance, a fight with a friend, a low score on a test, not getting selected to be on the school team or your parents saying no to a sleepover at your friend's place — all could be grounds for sadness.

Depression on the other hand seemed to feel more intense — a feeling that would come from the inside and have a life of its own. You could wake up feeling low and not want to get out of bed. There might not be any immediate reason or trigger for this. Going to school might become a major drag. You find you really need to push yourself to do things.

While feeling sadness is an essential part of living our lives, depression seems to be getting in the way of our lives.[64] Depression can be mild, severe, brief or long-lasting.

How do you deal with your sadness? It's not a very popular emotion — most of us want to get rid of it. When we are sad don't we have people coming and telling us to cheer up like it was some sort of an instant switch. Why is it not okay to feel this feeling? This reminds me of the image of sadness in the movie *Inside Out*. She is depicted as a blue, dull, boring character, with a voice that drags joy down … someone you wish would be gone.

The thing to remember is that without feeling sadness, we wouldn't be able to experience joy. Getting rid of sadness would also mean getting rid of joy and this would lead to feeling nothing. When we squish our feelings (whether it's sadness, anger, excitement or fear) or repress or deny them, we could be building on to depression.

Another misunderstood emotion is anger. Anger is often seen as our enemy with its destructive elements. Anger is, in fact, a very beautiful and powerful emotion. It can help motivate us to change aspects of our lives and it can also help us to advocate for ourselves. It has unfortunately earned a bad reputation because of how it seems to be responsible for our aggressive and violent acts. That's often a result of not learning how to adequately express our anger. We can express our anger in non-violent means of communication. It is, in fact, when we are unable to express our anger towards others that we tend to turn it against ourselves and it begins to 'chip away at us' from within. It becomes the inner critical voice that is fuelled by guilt and lack of self-worth. This unacknowledged anger can play a big role in depression.

The bottom line is, whatever age we are at, it's important that we learn to feel our feelings without judging ourselves.

AFFIRMATIONS FOR SELF

- Feel your feelings
- All your feelings are welcome and valid
- It's okay to reach out for help

RISK FACTORS FOR DEPRESSION

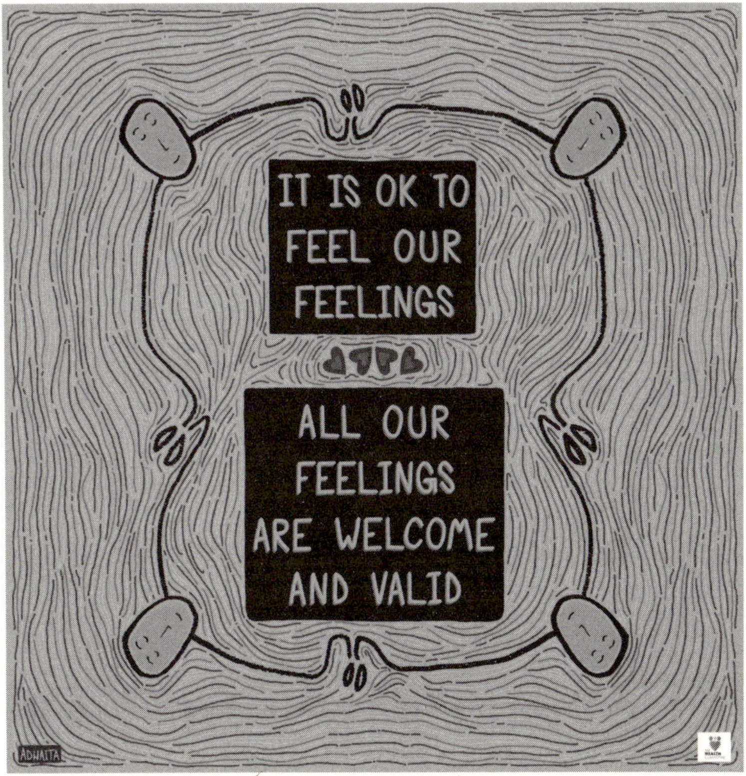

Artist: Adwaita Das

What are the factors that may lead to developing depression? There are certain risk factors that seem to increase the chances that a child or adolescent may develop depression such as:

- History of depression in a parent or sibling
- Family dysfunction or conflict with a caregiver
- Exposure to early adversity (such as abuse, neglect, the loss of a loved one in early life)
- Problems with friends or school/bullying
- Negative outlook or poor coping skills
- History of anxiety disorders, learning disabilities, attention deficit hyperactivity disorder, or significant defiance or conduct problems
- History of brain injury or low birth weight
- Chronic medical illness

TREATMENT OF DEPRESSION

A majority of adolescents in India, who are at risk for depression, do not receive treatment or receive it when the illness has become entrenched and chronic.[65]

Early intervention during childhood and adolescence can prevent depression from becoming full blown. Depression is a treatable condition. If you see any of the symptoms (listed earlier) it is advisable to consult a psychiatrist for an evaluation. There are two main forms of treatment, pharmacotherapy or drug therapy and psychological therapies.

PHARMACOTHERAPY OR DRUG THERAPY

Although psychotherapy is a major component in the treatment of childhood and adolescent depression, the use of medication is sometimes appropriate and is done by a psychiatrist. The medical professional takes into consideration the severity

and history of depression before initiating antidepressant therapy, i.e., treating depression with anti-depressant medication.[66] Do not attempt to prescribe or purchase medication without a proper prescription from a trained psychiatrist.

PSYCHOLOGICAL THERAPIES FOR CHILD AND ADOLESCENT DEPRESSION

COGNITIVE BEHAVIOUR THERAPY (CBT): CBT and interpersonal therapy have been proven effective in the treatment of adolescent depression, and CBT has been proven effective in the treatment of childhood depression. [67]

FAMILY THERAPY: Research findings suggest family therapy may be more effective for younger children with depression and for those whose mothers are depressed.[68]

MINDFULNESS-BASED COGNITIVE THERAPY (MBCT): Research studies have shown that practicing mindfulness help protect against the onset of depression as mindfulness practices aid affect regulation, i.e., being able to regulate your emotions and it also promotes self-acceptance. [69]

Mindfulness training in therapy can reduce self-reported rumination, depression and psychological distress. [70]

MBCT was shown to be as effective as antidepressants in preventing relapses of depression and allowed many subjects to discontinue medication.[71]

PARENTING A CHILD WITH DEPRESSION

It is challenging to parent a child who is suffering from depression. This can take a toll on you and there are times that you will find yourself feeling helpless, overwhelmed and anxious.

1. PARENT–CHILD COMMUNICATION cannot be over-emphasised. Giving your child a safe space lends an opportunity for them to be able to share their personal issues with you.

According to a study done in India on anxiety among high school students, it was found that a substantial proportion of adolescents perceived they did not receive quality time from fathers (32.1 per cent) and mothers (21.3 per cent). A large number of them also did not feel comfortable to share their personal issues with their parents (60.0 per cent for fathers and 40.0 per cent for mothers).[72]

Besides having regular conversations, it is crucial to understand how to respond to your child, especially when they are distressed. This helps build trust and you must let them know that they can come to you no matter what the difficulty.

STAYLISTENING, a tool developed by Patty Wipfler from her book *Listen* is simple and yet powerful, when used with children and adolescents[73].

- As the term suggests you stay and listen all the way through your child's distress.
- When you 'Staylisten', you move away from fixing things: instead you trust your child will recover and figure it out.
- You move away from lecturing, you assist your child as she clears away her upset.
- You sail with your child through her emotionally stormy seas.

Staylistening helps ease the parent's mind with respect to setting reasonable limits and also helps the child know that you are on their side. This tool can be especially helpful to facilitate supportive communication with your child when they are depressed.

When your child is depressed you can use staylistening as a tool, however, it's important that you are supportive and engaged with your child.

2. HOW CAN YOU BE SUPPORTIVE TO YOUR CHILD?

- You can work on strengthening your relationship by being empathetic. You can say, 'I am sorry you are going through this, I can imagine how hard it must be for you,' or, 'I am here for you,' 'I love you'.
- You can validate their emotions by reflecting their thoughts and emotions back to them. When your child is missing school and you say, 'It must be really hard for you to go to school when you are feeling so low,' you are validating the emotion, not the behaviour that could be unhelpful.
- You can be compassionately curious, and say, 'I know you have been feeling down lately, what would help you go to school?'

3. FOCUS ON THE EXCEPTIONS. There is a form of psychotherapy called solution-focused therapy that works on identifying exceptions to problems and elaborates on how we can do more of what helps. Noticing what your child can do rather than not is helpful. Parents with their best intentions in mind may still sound critical to their children. I have children often telling me that their parents remind them on a daily basis of what they haven't done: 'Why haven't you cleaned your room?' or, 'You didn't finish your meal?' or, 'Why haven't you finished your homework just yet?'

4. Most importantly, **TAKE CARE OF YOURSELF**. It's important to fuel your energy, take breaks, and have time with your partner and friends. Do not hesitate to reach out for support for yourself — you are not alone in this.

TOOL BOX FOR DEPRESSION

MINDFULNESS AND DEPRESSION: Mindfulness informed psychotherapy is gaining prominence as an effective evidence-based approach in the field of mental health. It is important to note that mindfulness alone is seldom enough for effective treatment of depression. It is usually a part of a multi-pronged approach.

So what is mindfulness? It is the awareness of the present experience with acceptance. There are mindfulness practices twhich assists in facing and thus help build affect tolerance (being able to tolerate intense emotions) and self-acceptance.

CULTIVATING KINDNESS AND SELF-COMPASSION: A valuable set of practices for treating depression involves cultivating self-compassion.[74] This is at the core of working towards self-acceptance and love.
It can be a powerful tool when used for self and the other.

I adapted this practice traditionally meant for the individual to the 'parent-child' dyad. I use it in my sessions if it seems appropriate. The families can then choose to practice it at home if they find it helpful.

This mindfulness practice has two parts to it — the first is for the parent to convey their love and blessings to their child. The second is for their child, who in return receives this love and gives it to back to themselves.

TOOL#1: 'PARENT-CHILD: LOVING KINDNESS MEDITATION'

In this exercise the child and parent sit face to face in a comfortable position looking at each other. Allowing the body and mind to settle with a few deep breaths.

- The parent holds or touches the hand of their child in whichever way that feels comfortable for the child — the parent then, not only with their attention but with loving attention, connects with their child and shares their warmth through their touch.
- With this loving attention the parent repeats softly and gently to the child, allowing the significance of their words to resonate with their heart:

May you be safe,
May you be peaceful,
May you be healthy,
May you live with ease.

(The parent can add any additional blessings they want for the child either spontaneously, or prepare them beforehand.)

- The child then repeats this for themselves by putting their hand on their own heart — with the loving attention that they have received, repeating softly and gently to themselves, allowing the significance of their words to resonate with their heart:

May I be safe,
May I be peaceful,
May I be healthy,

May I live with ease.

(The child can add any additional blessings for themselves if they want spontaneously, or prepare them beforehand.)

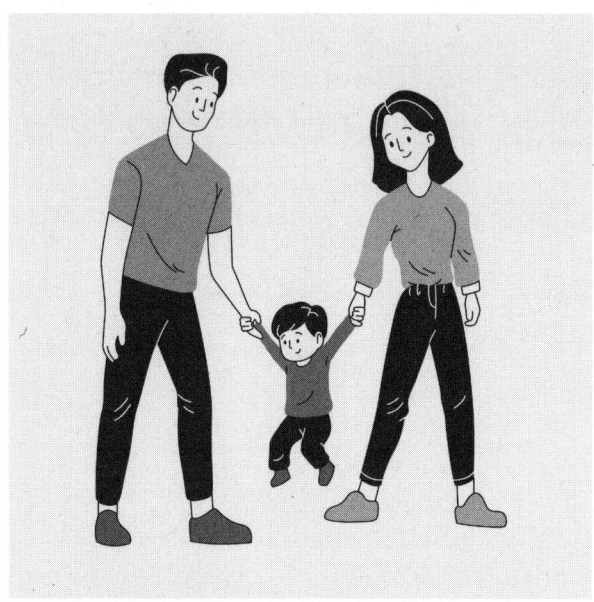

TOOL #2: MOOD TRACKER

• It can be helpful to keep a track of moods through the day or week. This information helps understand what factors such as time of day, situation, people, might be affecting the individual's moods.

- Rating scales can be used. 1–10 with 1 being awful and 10 being great.
- A review at the end of the week can help highlight any trends or triggers that you may have noticed. It also helps to identify the factors that were helpful when moods were good/ great.

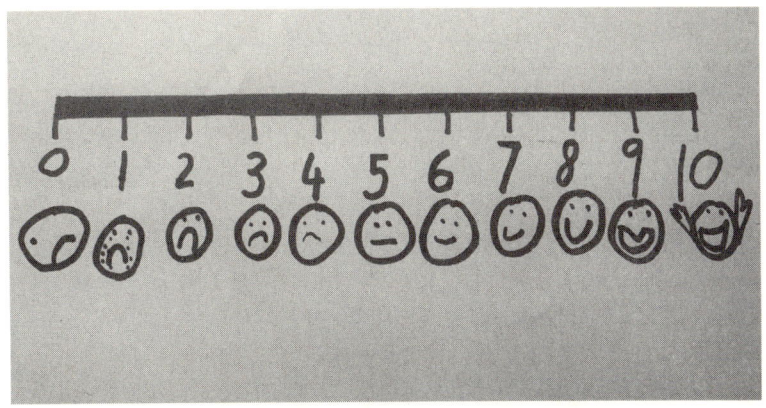

Mood Tracker by Nithanth Alva

TOOL#3: SUPPORT CIRCLES

- On a chart you can either draw or print concentric circles.
- Write your name in the middle and keep adding names of people you can talk to if you have a problem, i.e., people who care about you in each of the concentric circles.
- You can add as many people you wish to in each circle.
- The idea is to have a visual reminder that you are not alone and that you have people who you can reach out to.

CASE ILLUSTRATION: DEPRESSION AND MINDFULNESS-BASED THERAPY*

*Names and all identifying details have been changed to protect the privacy of individuals

Divya, a 16-year-old girl had just finished her 10th class Board exams and had reported that she was depressed. She was full of regret and disappointment for not having done well. She believed she wasn't a good student, she felt she hadn't worked hard enough and had wasted the academic year. She referred herself to a therapist.

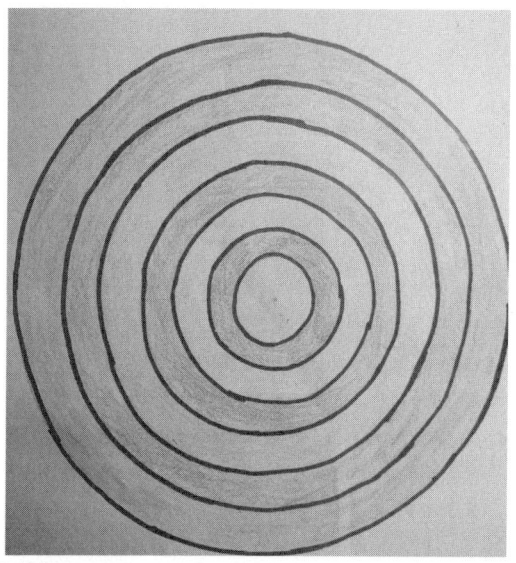

Support Circles by Manini Alva

REFLECTIONS:

- The therapist, informed by the mindfulness approach, asked her not to focus on the thought of 'not being good enough' but to pay attention to where she felt it in her body. She was able to identify points of heaviness in her head at the temples and this made her want to hang her head down. It felt like a burden — her head heavy with the painful thoughts of her not being worthy. As she hung her head down she was weeping and sharing how ashamed she was of letting her parents down.
- The therapist explored the possibility that the negative thoughts of how she wasn't 'good enough' were arising from her sadness and disappointment of having let herself and her parents down and perhaps it was not an accurate assessment of her skills as a student.

Questions that can help direct the mindfulness based process:

- Can you see that as just a thought? Instead of 'I am not good enough', you could say 'I am having the thought that I am not good enough.'
- Can you remember a time when you didn't think this way?

- Can you move below the level of thought into your feelings and physical sensations?

While for Divya the thought of not being 'good enough' was not just a thought, it was something the she believed in strongly and had internalised. The therapist worked with her through the mindfulness approach, as she found it helpful and combined it with family therapy work.

YOUNG ANXIETY

IS THIS 'NORMAL' ANXIETY?

Some anxiety is a normal aspect of development. Toddlers experience separation anxiety when they are separated from their mothers, fear of thunder, lightning, fire, darkness, nightmares are common in two to three year olds.

Five to seven year olds can be scared of specific objects (animals, ghosts, monsters), natural disasters, and, in fact, commonly have school anxiety. Older children and adolescents often become anxious and fear rejection from their peers.

Such difficulties should not be viewed as evidence of a disorder. However, if manifestations of anxiety become so exaggerated that they greatly impair functioning or cause severe distress then it should be taken seriously.

Parents need to be vigilant to see the difference between what seems to be the normal worries of childhood and what might seem like signs that require professional support. A good indicator would be when you find that your child is feeling overwhelmed and 'stuck' to the point where the anxiety starts coming in the way of them doing their normal day-to-day activities such as going to school, playing, falling asleep, or trying new things.

Additionally, with older children and adolescents, you need to be concerned if you notice sleep disturbances, panic episodes (trembling, sweating, shortness of breath, stomachaches, or headaches), obsessive thoughts or compulsive behaviour.

Children can experience feeling overwhelmed and 'stuck' in such situations.

Parents need to look out for when their anxiety starts coming in the way of doing normal daily functions like going to school, playing, falling asleep, or trying new things. Parents need to be vigilant to this difference between what seem to be the worries of childhood and what might seem like signs that can actually develop into an anxiety disorder if unattended to with professional support.

Childhood and adolescence is the core risk phase for the development of symptoms and syndromes of anxiety that may range from transient mild symptoms to full-blown anxiety disorders. [75]If you are concerned please schedule an appointment with a therapist. It is advisable to address such concerns at the earliest.

WHAT TO LOOK OUT FOR?

REFUSAL TO GO TO SCHOOL

Refusal to go to school is one of the most common instances of an anxiety disorder in children and adolescents. It's not that they fear school but this could be a result of separation anxiety, or social anxiety, or that child could also be avoiding school because of bullying issues. Bullying issues need to be taken seriously and systemic intervention, i.e., having the family and school work hand in hand is critical in supporting the child and stopping the bullying episodes.

There could also be other reasons for school refusal such as distress at home where there is conflict between the parents and the child stays at home to support one of the parents who may be leaning on them (unconsciously) for support. Family therapy can be very helpful in such cases.

COMPLAINS DIRECTLY ABOUT THEIR ANXIETY

- 'I am worried that I will never see you again' (separation anxiety)
- 'I am worried the kids will laugh at me' (social anxiety disorder)
- 'I cannot go to school because I have a stomach ache' (discomfort in terms of somatic complaints)

Do not dismiss or minimise your children's complaints. They are often telling the truth because an upset stomach, nausea and headaches can develop in children with anxiety. Several long-term follow-up studies[76] confirm that many children with regular somatic complaints, especially abdominal pain, have an underlying anxiety disorder.

To illustrate with an example, there was a 12-year-old child who had recurrent headaches, stomach aches and nausea. She would become anxious in situations where she might be far from a restroom and would thus refuse to leave her home. Her avoidance of social situations could, in turn, increase her anxiety when she anticipates or is forced to engage in activities outside the home. Here we see both school refusal and social anxiety as manifestations of her anxiety in addition to her somatic complaints.

There are many different types of anxiety disorders, including generalised anxiety, social anxiety, separation anxiety, obsessive-compulsive symptoms, phobias and panic. All of these disorders cause significant distress and a reduced level of functioning and competency for children and adolescents.

With reference to the DSM-5[77], here are the symptoms to look out for when checking for Generalised Anxiety Disorder (GAD), which is when an individual has excessive anxiety and worry about a variety of topics, events or activities. Worry occurs more often than not for at least six months and is clearly excessive. Please see this as indicative and do not attempt to self-diagnose or diagnose anyone on your own. Please consult with an expert if you have any concerns.

• The worry is experienced as very challenging to control. The worry in both adults and children may easily shift from one topic to another.
• The anxiety and worry are accompanied with at least three of the following physical or cognitive symptoms (In children, only one symptom is necessary for a diagnosis of GAD):
- Edginess or restlessness
- Tiring easily; more fatigued than usual
- Impaired concentration or feeling as though the mind goes blank
- Irritability (which may or may not be observable to others)
- Increased muscle aches or soreness
- Difficulty sleeping (due to trouble falling asleep or staying asleep, restlessness at night, or unsatisfying sleep)

RISK FACTORS: ANXIETY

In the etiology of anxiety disorders there is a complex interplay of biological and genetic vulnerabilities, temperamental qualities, negative environmental influences and negative attachment experiences, parental psychopathology, and disadvantageous socio-cultural factors.[78]

According to a paper 'Risk Factors of Anxiety Disorders in Children' by Malgorzata Dabkowska and Agnieszka Dabkowska-Mika,[79] biological risk factors include genetics and child temperament. Studies of environmental risk factors in the development of childhood anxiety disorders have focused on parent-child interactions and parental anxiety.

TREATMENT

Anxiety disorders in children and adolescents are treated with psychological therapies and drug or pharmacotherapy therapy.

PSYCHOLOGICAL THERAPIES INCLUDE:

• BEHAVIOURAL THERAPY: Cognitive behaviour therapy (CBT) is well regarded as an effective evidence-based treatment for childhood anxiety disorders. CBT has several key components: psycho education of child and caregivers regarding the nature of anxiety; techniques for managing somatic reactions identifying and challenging anxiety provoking thoughts; practicing problem-solving for coping with anticipated challenges; systematic exposure to feared situations or stimuli, including imaginal, simulated and in vivo methods, with special focus on desensitization to feared stimuli; and relapse prevention plans[80].

• MINDFULNESS BASED THERAPY: In the last decade, there has been growing research exploring the efficacy of mindfulness based treatments for anxiety disorders. In a recent study, mindfulness based therapy has shown significant reductions in anxiety and depressive symptoms across a wide range of presenting problems.[81]

The mindfulness approach focuses on:

- Expanding our awareness of experience
- Noticing reactions as to what they are and allowing them to be
- Developing kindness and compassion towards ourselves
- And intentionally choosing to engage in activities that matter to us as alternative ways of responding that can be cultivated through mindfulness practice.[82]

...

Now you may be wondering ... isn't worry just part and parcel of the modern experience?

Do you think it is normal to fear? Is fear a sign of weakness? Does worrying help us in any way? Wouldn't it be strange not to worry if things are amiss? There's nothing modern about worry, after all. During the Stone Age, cavemen feared the dark. Naturally, without light they couldn't see the predators that might have been lurking around them — this 'fear' protected them from stepping into the dark and getting killed. We are hard-wired to experience fear to help us survive. However, this also means that we may feel fear when we perceive the slightest threat. Some of us still fear the dark even in the safety of our homes with no real threat around. Our brains are naturally programmed to respond this way.

We do live in a frightening world — just reading the papers in the morning can be anxiety inducing — from terrorist attacks, to people dying in accidents, suicides, murders, abductions, a virus pandemic ... no wonder we are anxious.

Worrying becomes a way in which we are able to cope with life's unexpected threats and misfortunes. Worrying gives us the feeling that by thinking about situations or problems, we might be able to actively do something about them. This may be helpful at times when we are re-thinking a problem and are able to come up with alternatives. But at other times, worrying makes us even more anxious — for instance if you are stuck in traffic on the way to a movie, there is absolutely nothing you can do to get to your destination and worrying doesn't really help.

Now when worry turns into anxiety that becomes a regular feature in your life, it is helpful to get to know it better. Try to befriend your anxiety — you could try these exercises in the tool box to help you identify what triggers it, how it manifests itself and how it affects you.

TOOL BOX FOR ANXIETY

TOOL # 1: THOUGHT CLOUDS

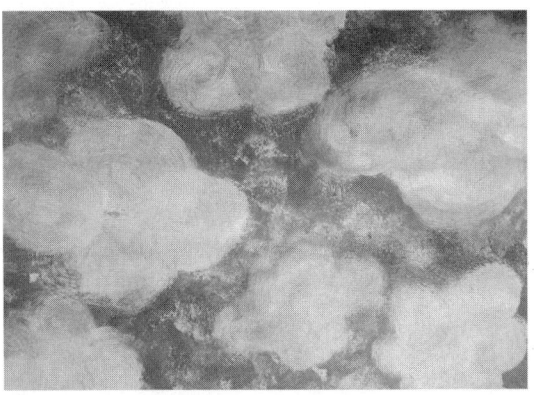

Thought Clouds by Manini Alva

This is a mindfulness exercise that we can try during times when we feel stuck in our thoughts.

'Thoughts are just thoughts' — they do not define us. So the metaphor of seeing thoughts as clouds helps to see them as transient, light and moving. So with the soft movement of these clouds our thoughts too pass by without staying stuck, relieving us of the anxiety that comes with it.

Find a comfortable position. You could either sit or lie down. Close your eyes if it is comfortable, and begin to notice what is going on inside of your body. Then slowly focus on your breath and do a few rounds of inhaling and exhaling. You could begin the imagery once you feel a little centred.

Imagine your thoughts are like the clouds passing through the sky — 'you' are not these 'thoughts' rather 'you' are awareness itself — 'you' are the sky.

As your thoughts arise, notice them ... label them as you would when you see different-shaped clouds as a kid! Children are able to quite quickly see all sorts of shapes, 'This one looks like a dragon' while this other cloud looks like a person's face ... similarly you could notice some thoughts are scary, sad, happy or meaningless ... let them pass ... the idea is that you can let them go and so they don't hold any power over you.

TOOL #2: GROUNDING TECHNIQUE 5-4-3-2-1

After a trauma if you find yourself having flashbacks and anxiety episodes you could try grounding techniques that can help control these symptoms temporarily by turning the attention away from the associated thoughts, memories, or worries, and refocusing on the present moment.

Using the 5-4-3-2-1 technique, you will purposefully take in the details of your surroundings using each of your senses. Strive to notice small details that your mind would usually tune out, such as distant sounds, or the texture of an ordinary object.

• What are **5** things you can see? Look for small details such as a pattern on the ceiling, the way light reflects off a surface, or an object you never noticed.

• What are **4** things you can feel? Notice the sensation of clothing on your body, the sun on your skin, or the feeling of the chair you are sitting on. Pick up an object and examine its weight, texture, and other physical qualities.

• What are **3** things you can hear? Pay special attention to the sounds your mind has tuned out, such as a ticking clock, distant traffic, or trees blowing in the wind.

• What are **2** things you can smell? Try to notice smells in the air around you, like an air freshener or freshly mowed grass. You may also look around for something that has a scent, such as a flower or an unlit candle.

• What is **1** thing you can taste? Carry gum, candy, or small snacks for this step. Pop one in your mouth and focus your attention closely on the flavours.

TOOL #3: EXTERNALISING YOUR WORRY

This is a classic narrative therapy technique for creating change. 'The problem is the problem, the person is not the problem' is an oft-quoted maxim of narrative therapy.

• When a problem has taken over someone to such an extent that they feel identified with it, it is useful to externalise it. This helps make it tangible and something that can be managed. You begin to develop a better understanding with your worries in this case and perhaps at some point are able to even befriend it.

- Method: You can externalise your worry by drawing it, writing about it, talking about it, singing about it — you can get as creative as you want — this helps approach it in a playful way.
- Questions you can ask: how does it look/feel/ taste? Does it have a name? What is its colour? What does it look like?

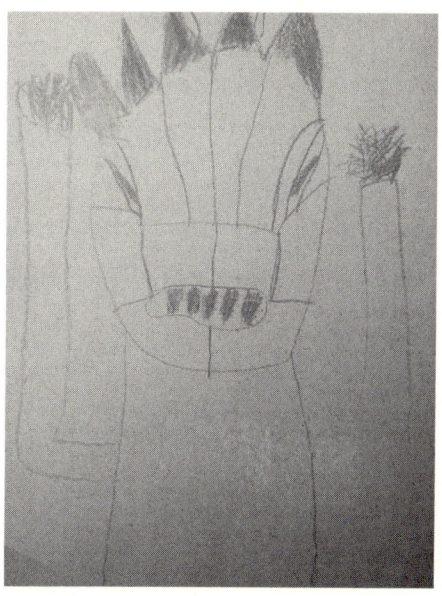

Image by Nithanth Alva

...

PARENTING AN ANXIOUS CHILD

Anxious children often have anxious parents. According to a study done on childhood anxiety, as many as 65 per cent of children of parents with anxiety disorders meet the criteria for an anxiety disorder.[83]

Since there is a high correlation between parent anxiety and child anxiety, parental support is instrumental in helping children manage and overcome their anxiety.

Here are some suggestions for parents:

• MANAGE NOT ELIMINATE: If your child is chronically anxious, instead of trying to eliminate the anxiety you could help him manage it more effectively. As a parent you will not be able to remove the triggers present, however you can help your child feel more supported as they face an anxiety-provoking situation.

I would like to share a personal instance of how I tried to manage a terrifying dental situation with my daughter. I know I am not in the minority when I say I fear dentists. Most grown adults do feel petrified at the thought of a dentist performing a root canal. My daughter needed to get braces and was very uncomfortable even at the thought of visiting a dentist. I found myself transferring my anxiety to her, which didn't help at all. Since I recognised my anxiety was coming in the way, I made it a point to ask my husband to accompany her on all her appointments. This was a good decision on my part. My husband, who seems unusually calm in dental situations, prepared her in advance before the visits and voila! She had a really good experience on her next dental visit. It also helped that we vetted the doctor and found someone who was very gentle and good with children. I understood quite clearly from this experience that trying to eliminate either my anxiety or my daughter's was not realistic, but managing the situation to make it less anxiety

provoking was helpful.

- VALIDATE YOUR CHILD'S FEELINGS. This does not mean that you are encouraging her anxious behaviour. When a child is anxious they are not feeling safe. When you empathise with how your child feels, she feels safe with you and trusts you to help her with her fears.

I find that instead of validating, most often parents with all good intentions to reduce the anxiety, try to:

- Minimise: For example, when a child is starting at a new school and expresses that she is anxious, you say, 'You've already moved two schools, it's not a big deal this time!'
- Negate: For example, when a child cries in fear of the doctor giving him an injection, you say, 'No, this injection will not hurt you! There's nothing for you to feel so scared about!'
- Shame the child: For example, when your son doesn't want to walk near the gutter because he is scared of the rats that might come out, saying something like, 'How can such a big boy be scared of such a small thing?'

Now, here's what you could say that would be more validating and supportive to your child's fear:

When a child is starting at a new school and expresses that she is anxious: 'Although you have moved two schools in the past, it's never easy going to a new one, I understand how anxious you must be about your first day.'

When a child cries in fear of the doctor giving him an injection: 'I know it looks big and scary and it will hurt you a little bit — would you like to hold my hand while the doctor gives you the injection?'

When your son doesn't want to walk near the gutter because he is scared of the rats that might come out: 'I know you are scared of rats, they can be quite gross sometimes — would you like to walk on the other side of the road with me?'

HERE ARE SOME DO'S AND DON'TS:

DON'T ASK LEADING QUESTIONS: Be curious about your child's feelings and ask open-ended questions.

Instead of, 'Are you anxious about going to your new school tomorrow?' or, 'Are you worried about the upcoming maths exam?' … you could ask, 'How are you feeling about your first day at your new school?' or, 'How are you feeling about the upcoming exams?'

DON'T PRE-EMPT YOUR CHILD'S FEARS: Let's say your child had a bad experience in the pool. The next time you go swimming you may want to avoid saying, 'Do you think you might be scared of swimming because of what happened last time in the pool?' You may unintentionally give him the message that he needs to be anxious in the pool.

DO ENCOURAGE YOUR CHILD'S EFFORTS: As you find your child doing better around their anxiety triggers, appreciate even the smallest effort they make in tolerating the anxiety.

DO HAVE A PLAN: When children talk to their parents about their worst fears, having contingency plans help them feel less anxious. If your child's worst fears are that they would get lost in the metro during your trip, you can prepare a safety plan in advance. You can write your phone number on a piece of paper that they can keep it in their pocket, or you can have a rule about how they need to get off at the next station and wait near the closest security booth in case you get separated. Having a plan helps reduce anxiety for some children.

DO WORK ON YOUR OWN ANXIETY — GET SUPPORT: Children will learn to cope with their anxiety as they watch you cope with yours. While you cannot always be perfectly calm and anxiety free, seeing you meditate, taking time off or talking to a friend for support gives them the assurance that their parents seem to have a grip on things.

CHILD SEXUAL ABUSE (CSA)

The World Health Organization (WHO) defines Child Sexual Abuse (CSA) as 'the involvement of a child in sexual activity that he or she does not fully comprehend, is unable to give informed consent to, or for which the child is not developmentally prepared and cannot give consent, or that violates the laws or social taboos of society.' CSA includes an array of sexual activities like fondling, inviting a child to touch or be touched sexually, intercourse, exhibitionism, involving a child in prostitution or pornography, or online child luring by cyber-predators.

With an increase in awareness and advocacy around child protection, the Government of India passed 'The Protection of Children from Sexual Offences (POCSO)' law in 2012. This act criminalises a range of acts, including rape, harassment, and exploitation for pornography involving a child below 18 years of age and mandates the setting up of Special Courts to expedite trials of these offences. There is a significant underreporting of CSA to authorities due to the prevalent taboo that still continues to be the reality of CSA in India.

According to the CHILDLINE India foundation[84], India has the world's largest number of sexually abused children: with a child below 16 years raped every 155 minutes, a child below 10 every 13 hours and one in every 10 children sexually abused at any point of time. A study done by the Union Ministry of Women and Child Development (WCD Ministry) also revealed that 53 per cent of the interviewed children reported having faced some form of sexual abuse and proved that boys were as vulnerable to abuse as girls.[85]

These statistics are overwhelming and bring with it the desperate urgency to initiate prevention and awareness programmes for our community.

WARNING SIGNS IN CHILDREN AND ADOLESCENTS OF POSSIBLE CHILD SEXUAL ABUSE:

- Acting out in an inappropriate sexual way with toys or objects
- Nightmares, sleeping problems
- Becoming withdrawn or very clingy
- Becoming unusually secretive
- Sudden unexplained personality changes, mood swings and seeming insecure
- Regressing to younger behaviours, for e.g., bedwetting
- Unaccountable fear of particular places or people
- Outburst of anger
- Changes in eating habits
- New adult words for body parts and no obvious source
- Talk of a new, older friend and unexplained money or gifts
- Self-harm (cutting, burning or other harmful activities)

- Physical signs, such as, unexplained soreness or bruises around genitals or mouth, sexually transmitted diseases, pregnancy
- Running away
- Not wanting to be alone with a particular child or young person

Please be aware that any one sign does not indicate sexual abuse, but it is the presence of several warning signs that alerts us that parents need to investigate this further and seek support. Some of the signs listed could also come up during other times of stress, such as when parents are going through a divorce or death of a family member, bullying issues at school or any other trauma that the child may have faced.

Please do raise any concerns with a trained counsellor or psychotherapist.

PHYSICAL WARNING SIGNS:

These physical signs are rare, however, if you see them your child needs immediate medical attention.

- Pain, discoloration, bleeding or discharges in genitals, anus or mouth
- Persistent or recurring pain during urination and bowel movements
- Wetting and soiling accidents unrelated to toilet training

IF A CHILD TELLS YOU ABOUT ABUSE:

Three quarters of children who are sexually abused do not tell anyone about it and many keep their secret all their lives. Sexual abusers are more likely to be people we know, and could well be people we care about; more than eight out of

Young
MENTAL HEALTH

10 children who are sexually abused know their abuser. They are family members or friends, neighbours or babysitters — many hold responsible positions in society. The closer the relationship between the abuser and the victim, the less likely they are to talk about it.

Children often show us rather than tell us that something is worrying or upsetting them so being aware of the warning sign is vital. However, children may give vague hints that something is happening. Their information may not be clear and they may not have the words to explain what is happening to them. The way adults respond to this is vital to ensuring the child's safety.

RESPOND WITH CARE AND URGENCY: If you think a child is trying to tell you about a sexually abusive situation, respond promptly and with care. In our Indian settings, unfortunately we don't feel safe enough to go to the police or social services as people in other countries would, however you can call a child helpline for guidance and it is highly recommended that you contact a mental health professional for support at the earliest.

BELIEVE THE CHILD: If a child trusts you enough to tell you about abuse, you must remember that they rarely lie about such things. Although it may be hard to believe that someone we trust or care about is capable of sexually abusing a child, it's highly unlikely that a child would deliberately make false accusations about sexual behaviours.

The pressures on the child to keep silent are enormous. It takes tremendous courage to talk about abuse. A child's claim that sexual abuse did not happen (when it actually did), or taking back a disclosure of abuse are common. Sometimes the child's account of what happened changes or evolves over time. This is a common pattern for disclosure and should not invalidate their story.

BE SUPPORTIVE: It is important that children feel supported — do not dismiss their claims or discourage them from talking about it.

STAY CALM: If they are talking to you about it, don't get angry or upset. Stay calm and steady. If you get angry the child may think you are going to punish them — this will play into the hands of the abuser who warned the child not to tell. If the child fears you will become upset or distressed they are less likely to disclose in order to protect you emotionally.

BE CARING: Make sure the child knows you love them and that they have done nothing wrong — and keep reminding them that. The child will need to see that adults believe them and they are doing all they can to protect them. Make sure the child knows they were right to talk about it and that you are glad they came to you.

FACE THE PROBLEM: When the abuse is known, adults must face the problem honestly, protect the child at all costs and place responsibility appropriately with the abuser.

RE-ESTABLISH SAFETY: Do what is necessary to protect the child from further harm. Put into place a family safety plan, you can do this with the therapist or with other members of the family. The family safety plan includes being aware of the risk factors (the factors that puts someone at risk of sexually abusing a child); physical factors, e.g., being in close proximity to a child; a situational risk factor, e.g., lack of parental oversight. However, alongside being aware of risk factors other protective factors — the things a family can do to keep the family safer — are important to be aware of and consider. Protective factors can include good communication within the family; supportive relationships; appropriate rules and boundaries. Such protective factors are the building blocks of your family and provide a good foundation for developing an effective family safety plan.

Seek professional help, therapists can guide you towards safety and healing.

DO NOT DESPAIR: Children can and do recover from child sexual abuse. It is incredibly difficult to hear that someone you love has been hurt in such a way but help to recovery is available.

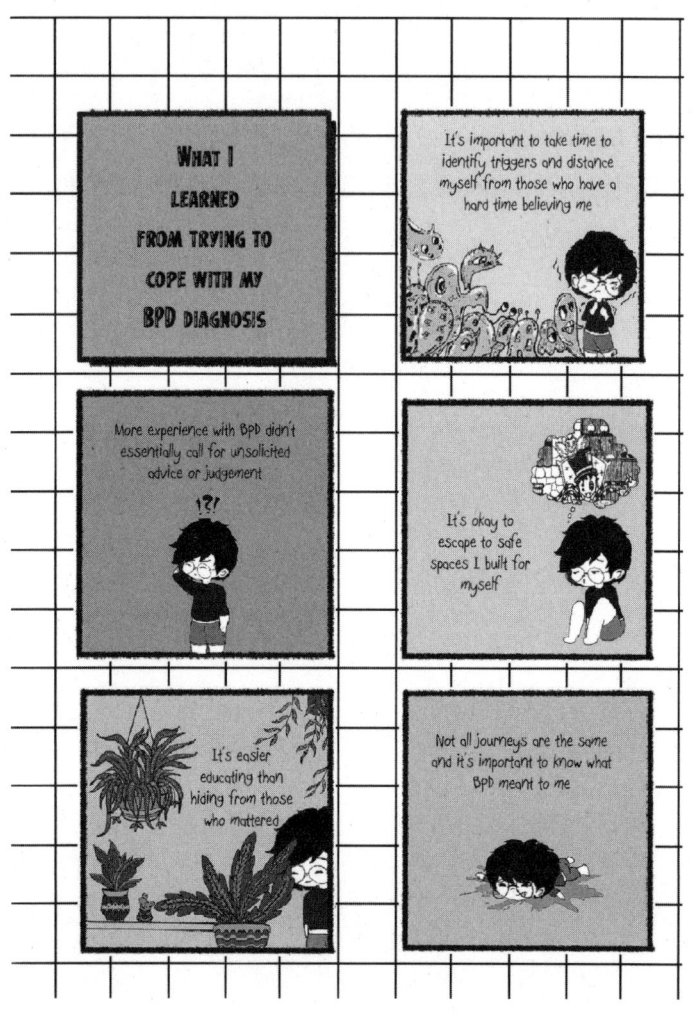

Chapter 16
IN THEIR OWN WORDS
What I Learned from Trying to Cope with my Borderline Personality Diagnosis: Story and Art by Solo

About the Artist: Solo is a writer and cartoonist from Bangalore. She likes reading, playing video games and binge-watching Netflix. Her life would have been rather unremarkable had it not been for her BPD-fuelled imagination. She also has four cats. Check out more work at stripteasethemag.com

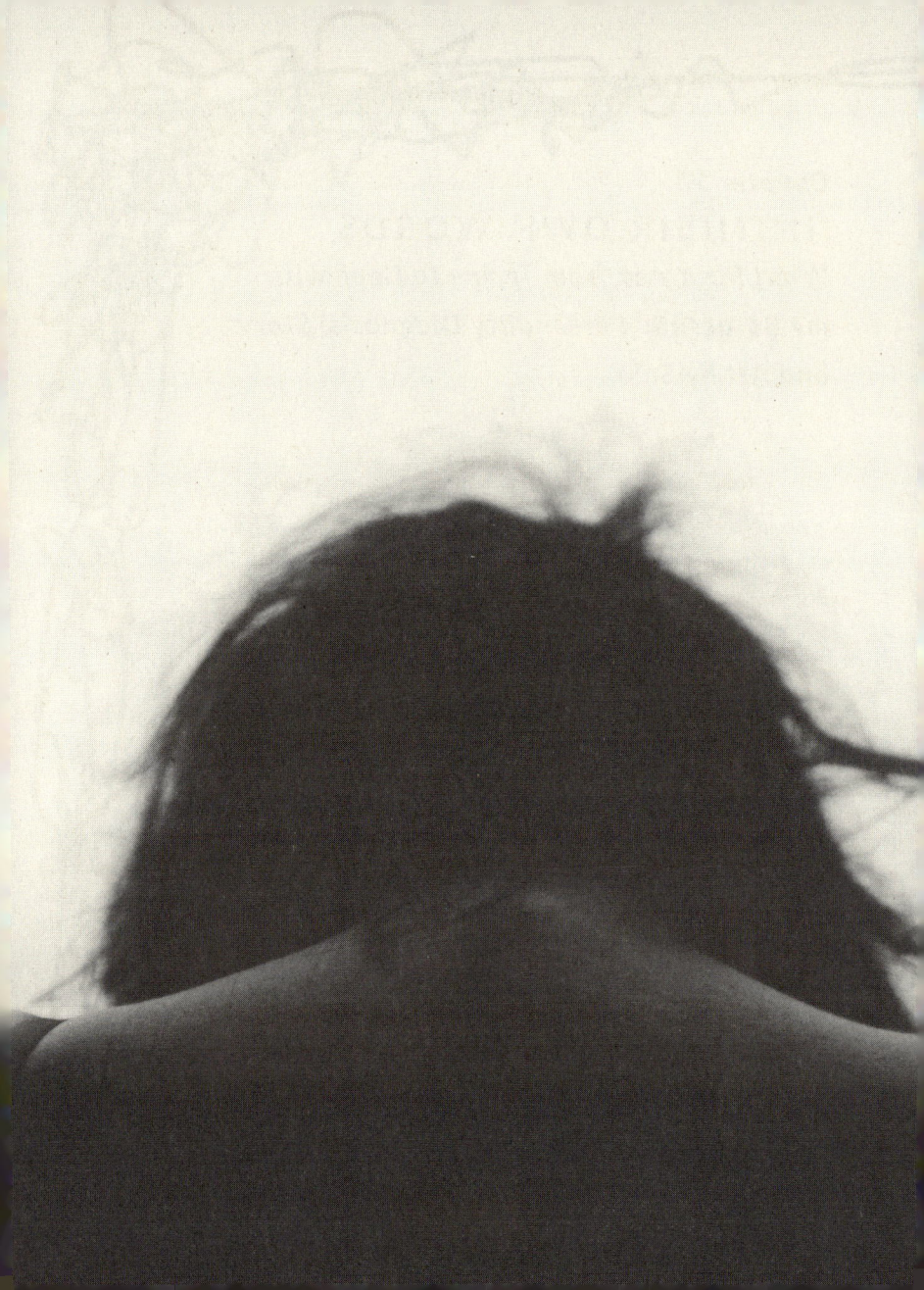

Chapter 17
IN THEIR OWN WORDS: OVERCOMING AN EATING DISORDER[86]
Anonymous

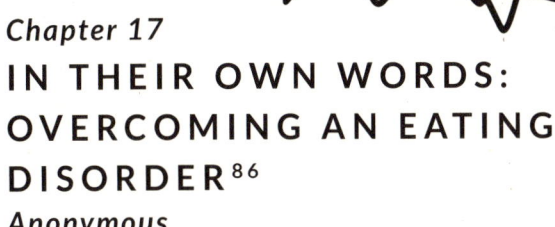

(Trigger Warning: Eating Disorder/Food Addiction)

'You're not fat, you're just big.'

This was a common refrain that I heard from my pre-teens till well into young adulthood. The various theories about deranged thyroid hormones to a heavy bone structure to the fact that the sinuses could be playing up offered little comfort. As time went on, the pants size only increased and the need to keep finding excuses as to why I was the way I was grew.

It wasn't always like this. I grew up as an energetic young boy who played and ran around more than most kids. I was thin in every sense of the word and enjoyed my time out in the open. Sports were a useful release for the excess energy and also helped me combat my occassionally debilitating habit of attention deficiency.

Then came a setback for a family member, which meant that my parents could not spend enough time with me once I got back from school. I was all of 10 years old and often felt lonely and alone. Paradoxically, the more I found myself alone, the more I wanted to be alone. It was then that I remember that my only solace would be food. Nothing in particular, but everything in general. I would eat my normal meals but would love to go out when possible to taste some of the more fattening stuff. Then the meal portions began to grow. For a child of my age, I was probably consuming that of a young adult. But I couldn't stop. I would feel the warm comfort of food taking some of the loneliness away. It was like a drug that made you feel better.

As things on the home front improved, I came back to a more normal routine. Only that normal by now meant over-eating three times a day. My doting mother, probably with a sense of guilt of having not spent enough time with me, fed us lovingly. At first, my weight gain was not obvious. Many pre-adolescents are heavier and tend to lose the excess fat as their bodies undergo the hormonal roller coaster that is adolescence.

Then one day it happened.

During the annual height and weight measurement that was mandatory as part of our school's physical education curriculum, I was amongst the tallest, but also amongst the heaviest. I was 13, nearly six feet tall and weighed close to 90 kgs. I remember how my classmates laughed with glee and childish meanness (that we thankfully lose with age) as they saw the needle on the scale move energetically towards the 90 kg mark. A few girls sniggered at the fact that I weighed as much as the two of them put together. The weight and how it looked on me ensured that a promising talent in swimming was given up and given a decent burial. I just could not stand the way people looked at me in the changing room. I was determined to let go of all situations where I would have to be in a changing room with other people. I took recourse to avoid rather than confront what was becoming increasingly clear and unsustainable.

While this shook my confidence on the inside, I was still a different person on the outside. Outgoing and gregarious, full of self-confidence, I took the weight in my stride. The only comfort came from food. Ironically, even more food. I remember the time when I was taken to restaurants and instead of asking for the food that no one ate to be packed, I polished it all off with a great sense of accomplishment. I would eat in between meals that were heavy to begin with. The 'this is how men must eat' bravado of some of the senior members of the family, gave me a false sense of everything being all right. They say you consume food, but in my case, the food consumed me.

There were dinners at home, when I would overhear friends of my parents refer to how much weight I had put on, and whether my parents intended to 'do something about it'. I remember my parents requesting their friends to not broach the subject because I was sensitive about the issue. This made me take to food even more, but with a subtle difference. In order to show how normal my eating habits were, I would consume a normal meal when in company, but as soon as I would retire to my room, I would look for food to eat and satiate my desire, which took the form of addiction. There was a time when I would hide food in my room, just so that I could have access to it when everyone was asleep, or when I was alone. I could not, at that stage in my life, differentiate between normal desires for nutrition and the occasional need to indulge, with that of what I was experiencing, the overwhelming need to satiate an unnatural appetite.

Slowly but steadily, by the time I was 16 years old, I weighed in at 110 kgs. It is no exaggeration to say that I could not find clothes of my size. These were not the

days when 'plus sizes' were acceptable. I had run through most of the men's sizes and the only option remaining was to go to wholesalers to find bigger sizes. With a shirt size of 46 and a waist size of 40, finding clothes became a task. This at a time when my friends had girlfriends and were looking at donning the latest in fashion. I, on the other hand, was looking for clothes to fit and someone to accept me for what I was.

The moment of truth, when it really hit me, was in a changing room in a men's clothing store. The cubicle with its functionality of ensuring privacy yet offering a closer look, did just that — only at a more profound psychological level. The trousers that I was trying on just did not fit. With tears in my eyes, I did not have the heart to go out and ask for a bigger size, knowing fully well that I would be the butt of all jokes amongst the salespeople. I took a long hard look at myself. This is not what I wanted to be. I did not want to be intricately linked and associated with being fat (or big or whatever). I did not want food to have a hold over me anymore. I knew that just as determined as I was to ensure that the snide remarks, the jeers and the innuendo about how I looked didn't affect me on the outside, I did not feel good on the inside.

I came out of the cubicle; quietly handed over the trousers to the salesman, making some perfunctory excuse about how it was not the shade I was wanted and told my parents to leave the store. I went home, locked myself up in the bathroom and cried. I didn't want to be this way anymore. Food had consumed me. It was the elixir that offered comfort but at a price. It was a price I wasn't willing to pay. I decided to do something that I had not done for years — I got onto a weighing scale myself. The needle finally stopped moving at 117 kgs. At 6 feet 2 inches and 18 years old, I was more than big — I was hurtling towards disaster.

It was time to change.

...

The New Year's Eve celebration was the biggest for all of a century — it was the day to enter a new millennium, not just a new year. The age of a new era, one paralysed at that time with the fear of the Y2K bug, was a time of hope and change. It was a time when I made a reappearance to the club where we used to go every New Year's Eve, ever since we were children. For the past few years I had stopped going. I just could not bring myself to. I felt that the whole world would be staring at this unnatural creation that was defying all laws of normalcy.

But this year was different. Dressed in a suit, and with old school friends, I made it to the club which was done up with its usual splendour, the customary DJ belting out hits, the sound of 'cheers' and small talk being drowned in the clink of glasses and the waft of sumptuous food. The first person I vaguely knew from school walked right past me. I thought she probably didn't see me so I kept walking, making my way to the centre of the gaiety. The second group of friends too walked past me and went straight to the other people I was with.

I hadn't met this lot ever since I had finished school, which was close to over a year now. As they spoke, a friend of mine pointed out to me and said, 'Why haven't you said hello?' That's when I saw a reaction that I hadn't seen before, which I became used to as the evening drew on. There was a collective gasp followed by a quick succession of 'ooh-ing' and 'aah-ing' by the group. 'My god, bro what happened to you?', 'You don't look the same, man!', 'You've shrunk!', 'You look good ya', 'How much weight have you lost — like 20 kgs?'

Young
MENTAL HEALTH

'No,' I said, '40 kilos.'

The proverbial penny dropped. I was the toast (whole wheat preferably) of the party. All was forgotten. The young ladies who sneered previously asked me for a dance. The now young men who (had) laughed, went about showing me off, as if they had accomplished something in my looking the way I did.

Maybe they did.

My mood elevated. The attention was tremendous and it did my confidence a whole lot of good. I was under 20 years of age, had gotten into medical school and most importantly, weighed 77 kilos.

The sense of being part of a once-shunned group made me feel accomplished. But it also taught me a valuable lesson. I felt the attention and my craving for it now as shallow. I realised that just the way I looked changed the way people saw me. I was still the same person, only in a new packaging! But I realised to the world that's what matters. It made me value my friends who had stuck with me through thick and thin (pun intended) even more. It made me look at those who had a newfound love for me — platonic and other variants — with a minor sense of disdain. All that matters is what you look like, not what you are within.

Writing back as I am now in my mid-30s, this realisation should have made me more ambivalent towards how I looked or weighed, to being more comfortable in my skin and being healthy. But when you are 20, 'acceptable' and wanting to make up for lost time, it had disastrous consequences. I became determined to ensure that I continue to look like I did the day we entered the year 2000, lest I go back to being shunned and shabby.

The journey from being an overweight teenager, unmindfully addicted to food, to one who was 'normal' was arduous. When I look back at what I did, I do feel a sense of accomplishment. I began slowly. It was something which was not going to be a flash in the pan. The reason was not so much as scientific enlightenment as the twin trouble of not being able to exercise beyond 20 minutes to begin with and not wanting anyone to find out.

Any time that I did refer to my wanting to lose weight or to start to exercise, friends would tell me that I shouldn't bother, 'Be yourself, everyone is unique,' and so on. My parents thought it was a good thing to do, but didn't really look sure if I would see the fad through. We had a lovely park at the back of the house. I began by walking gradually, a steady pace for 20 minutes every day. The result of this was increased hunger pangs. I decided that I must curb some this urge if I was to be realistic in what I wanted to achieve. My saviour came in the form of the simplest element known to man — water. I began drinking water like medicine. Gradually from a litre a day, it built up four times that amount. I started reading up on proteins, carbohydrates and concepts like Basal Metabolic Rate and such like. It helped.

Month on month, the weight started shedding. Gradually, the hunger pangs also abated. I reached a point when I became obsessed about not wanting to eat, but wanting to exercise incessantly. I walked more often that earlier. I began running on the treadmill and hitting the gym. The accelerated loss of weight hurtled on. In a year I lost over 30 kilos. The clothes stopped fitting and people began to notice a considerable difference in how I looked. I will never forget the day when I walked into the same clothing store — shunned out of self-shame a year ago — and buying clothes off the rack. The store salesman didn't recognise me. The biggest fillip in doing so was also to my mood. Gone was the gloominess of the past. A new cheery self-developed from within. As I got on with my routine and regime, I would

invariably hit plateaus — weeks and months would pass without the needle moving any further on the weighing scale. It was then that I would further reduce my food intake and exercise even more. Little did I realise that my aversion to food was becoming the new problem in my life. I went from an addiction to food … to being addicted to no food.

As the weight shed, my confidence grew and my attitudes changed as well. Regrettably, being overweight once did not make me empathetic towards people with a similar plight. I would often look at obese or oversight folk and wonder why they didn't do something about it. From complaining about being just a label — fat — for so many all my life, I began doing the same with others. But the biggest physical damage I did in this warped obsession with food and weight was to virtually starve myself of nutrition. It worked till the time the body and mind could hold up. It was a race to the bottom, but I was convinced that I could manage and that if I ate, I would become fat. Today, I look back and would neatly label that as anorexic behaviour. But a state of mind is not a label. It is a state. It is a being, an existence.

The inevitable did happen. My friends and I were out one evening. I remember not having eaten a solid meal for over 24 hours — a new normal for me. I looked gaunt, bones jutting with sunken eyes — but mentally feeling great at being 'thin'. I remember eating something along with the beer that I had ordered. Immediately, my heart began to race, I broke out into a cold sweat and a hazy curtain feel in front of my eyes. I shook myself up and drank a little water. I decided to head to the restroom to check what was wrong. As soon as I was in, I bent over the sink to wash my face. The next thing I remember was a few people hollering over me — throwing water to wake me up. I got up — dazed and confused (but still thin, thankfully). My friends had gathered around by then, being called out by the Good Loomaritans.

'Dude what happened?' I asked profoundly.
'You passed out!'
'Are you ok?'

I gave a vague yes and said I think I need some rest. I drove home and sat up till late at night wondering what and how it happened.

My aversion to food did not change. I would pick at my food, then drink enough liquids to keep me going and get through the day. Breakfast was meaningless and dinner best skipped. The medical school curriculum meant that lunch was a blink-and-miss-it experience. I never realised the damage I was doing to myself by doing what I was doing.

Then it happened again.

A second and a third fainting and blackout episode when I was out with friends and company meant that I decided going out was the problem.

I became averse to stepping out of the house — lest it happen again. The mild agoraphobia made me house-bound for a month. No one noticed because exams were on, so staying at home was the given thing. But deep inside I knew, stepping out of the house could be dangerous and embarrassing. I was scared still, period.

It was well after the exams got over that I had run out of excuses to not go out and meet people. I remember being terrified at the very thought of going out and meeting friends. I decided that I would not eat or drink. The evening was a dull but uneventful affair. I decided to concoct a story of how I had given up alcohol and therefore could not go out with my friends anymore. Deep inside, a gnawing reality began hitting me.

I was 23 had just become a doctor, managed to win a huge personal battle over food addiction and weight — and was now heading towards another 'man-made' crisis. It was time. I decided to confront the problem head-on. I decided to start becoming more aware of what was happening to me — physically, physiologically and psychologically, and more importantly try to understand why was it happening. I started reading on behaviours and attitudes, addictions and their origins. A basic textbook on Cognitive Behaviour Therapy was very useful. It offered simple yet effective techniques around thoughts, feelings and actions. Reading about people who battled afflictions helped to bring some sense of normalcy to what I was undergoing. But these were all time-consuming measures. CBT takes two to three months of daily practice to be effective.

Similarly, breaking old thoughts and habits is like effective exercise — it needs to be done daily. Changing one's outlook towards life, one's body image and to feel normal takes probably a lifetime. So while the acute problem has been addressed, the chronic is a work in progress.

It's been nearly a decade since I had to battle those demons.

Looking back at that time, I find some of it scary, some even funny, some fascinating and many instances upsetting. Has it made me a better, more balanced person? Yes. The biggest challenge life threw at me was to make me fat. It helped me understand myself and become a better person — in more ways than one. It helped me to explore the workings of the mind like no other experience could have.

I continue to weigh as much as a person of my size should. I exercise regularly,

have taken to naturopathy and organic foods and am happy with the way I look. I maintain a love–hate relationship with food, but it is more a friendly fight than a fight to the finish. I still am concerned about putting on weight, but don't feel it like an all-consuming fixation that will define my life. My friends still hold me up as an example of someone who battled weight issues and won over it. Many relatives refer to it as something in the distant past, which was a 'phase'. I have internalised it and moved on.

But what worries me is how we have moved as a society. There is more awareness on mental illness, body image, food addiction and other issues than at the turn of the century. But the progress is patchy and uneven. School children are not taught about body image, about what constitutes 'normal', about mental disease and what to do if you have issues.

Yes, we now find counsellors in most schools, but there needs to be a deeper integration of these issues into the curriculum itself. Reaching out for help on mental disease and addiction is still taboo and has many barriers. As a society and culture we are witnessing a stereotyping of what is a normal body type, glamourising size zero-ism and body shaming. Our selfie-obsessed culture means that teens and those who don't fit the stereotype are adopting means to hide as much as they show. We are ingraining a sense of normal and abnormal when no such thing exists. Conditions like anorexia, mood disorders, body dysmorphia and others are real. But they can be transitionary if managed and contextualised. We need to help arm people with the tools to fight the battle with themselves.

There is no greater accomplishment that winning over the self. And there is no better time than now.

(Editor's note: If you or a loved one suffer from an eating disorder, please do reach out for professional help)

UNDERSTANDING EATING DISORDERS AND BODY IMAGE DISORDERS

Like many issues, many of us take our lead from popular culture when it comes to eating disorders like bulimia or anorexia. More often than not, it's seen as a 'problem of privilege', and something to be sneered at. But living with an eating disorder is more common than you might think, though unfortunately, the subject seems to be under-researched in India[87], with a lack of accurate nation-wide statistics. For additional context and perspective though, here are some numbers to think about — the American National Eating Disorders Association estimates 20 million women and 10 million men in the USA will suffer an eating disorder at some stage of their lives.[88]

Globally, the prevalence is around 70 million people worldwide according to the National Eating Disorder Association.[89]

We asked a few mental health experts here in India for their take.

WHAT ARE EATING DISORDERS?

'Eating disorders (ED) are conditions when an individual engages in abnormal eating behaviours that negatively impacts the health, emotions and lifestyle behaviours. It affects an individual's physical and mental health, and can make the individual dysfunctional on a day to day level. Often, body image issues can arise from ED. Eating Disorders can include conditions like anorexia nervosa, bulimia, and binge disorders,' says Pragya Lodha, a Mumbai-based clinical psychologist and research associate at De Sousa Foundation and honorary associate editor of the Indian Journal of Mental Health and Programme Director of The MINDS Foundation.

COMMON EATING DISORDERS[90]

Anorexia nervosa: This is characterised by a persistent, even drastic restriction on food intake. This disorder includes an extreme fear of gaining weight; people can often have an unrealistic or distorted self-perception of weight and body size and shape.

Bulimia: This eating disorder is characterised by inducing vomiting or somehow 'purging' the system, usually after eating too much food, or 'binge-eating'. There is frequently a loss of control or sense of no control on the amount of food ingested. Other behaviours include use of laxatives or diuretics or fasting or over-exercising.

Binge-eating disorders: This is characterised by frequently eaten much larger-than-standard portions of food. Unlike with bulimia, there is no purging behaviour.

There are other eating disorders, and more information on many sites online, on the theories as to what leads to these disorders, which you might want to read about in more depth to be aware of any behaviour that might be symptomatic.

People bringing in loved ones, often use terms like 'depression', 'anxiety', 'not just eating well', or 'attention-seeking behaviour', says Smriti Joshi, lead psychologist Wysa, when asked about any colloquial terms used here in India. 'Individuals coming in themselves (for a consultation) often first come in reporting difficulties at work or at relationship or with managing their moods, or presenting an inability to eat more like a psycho-somatic complaint like: 'I don't know what happens when I eat, I just need to puke then' or 'pata nai khana dekh ke kya hota hai — *khaya hi nai jaata (I don't know what happens when I say food, I can't eat it)*'.

WHAT IS BODY IMAGE DISORDER?

Everyone has some sense of body image. It can be positive or negative, but essentially has to do with you how you perceive your own body, your own physical appearance.[91] A negative body image can lead to low self-esteem, depression, even eating disorders and can involve feelings of shame and low self-worth, as the US National Eating Disorders Association lists out on its site. [92]

'Body image concerns become a disorder when the concerns with body parts and appearances are irrational. The perception of very minor issues blows out of proportion by the individual and makes them dysfunctional. Anxiety and depressive features surface,' says Lodha.

'When body image issues are on an extreme level, where it becomes psycho-pathological, it is called Body Dysmorphic Disorder (BDD). BDD is the severe condition of having several and chronic body image issues. It explains concerns about body or body parts and appearance even when there is no problem or the problem is minor enough to cause any trouble. The preoccupation is to look perfect and there is a concern as to how others are perceiving the person,' she adds.

Lodha shares more information from her experience.

'Eating disorders and body image issues are seen very commonly, especially so in the younger cohort, say, between ages 14–25/27 years broadly.[93] Most often people don't come in for therapy for these two concerns but it presents as anxiety and depression almost always. These are concerns that usually don't get labelled as primary problems. Meaning, people may come with primary concerns of lack of confidence, low self-esteem, inability to work, inability to maintain relationships —

which often has body image issues as underlying reasons.'

'It is most often seen in females but sometimes is also seen in males. Females present with anorexia nervosa and bulimia and ED is also sometimes seen with a need to maintain a certain weight, appear a certain way or to be able to be "fit" enough to wear certain kinds of clothes.' But she adds some more perspective, 'It is common to see body building addiction in males which also often is accompanied by abnormal eating habits, over-consumption of protein shakes, starving and excessive focus on muscle-building.'

'Eating disorders and body image issues or BDD may not always present as full-blown disorders but fundamentally are seen far more in younger people. Additionally, a lot of people with BDD often go to cosmetologists rather than come to us (psychotherapists and psychiatrists) since they are convinced that there is a flaw that needs to be corrected, versus this being a presentation of anxiety (and/or sometimes other neurotic or severe mental states as well).'

Are there additional concerns with many of us buying into the projected perfection of online personas, concerns that go beyond the filters we use to make ourselves conform to socially sanctioned ideals of beauty? You bet.

'ED and body image issues are also very commonly seen among younger girls aspiring to have appearances like models; it is also sometimes seen as one's ability to be desirable enough as a partner, very common to see younger people feeling validated with their social media profiles looking the best and thus striving for better profiles by engaging in abnormal and inadequate eating, starving, preoccupations with body appearances. Recently, TikTok has been in controversy,[94] regarding promoting eating disorders due to the inability to screen for people posting on pro-

anorexia TikToks — though some measures have been taken, it has been reported to have triggered many globally.'

Like Joshi, Lodha agrees that there are no colloquial terms in common parlance in India when it comes to eating disorders or body image issues, but shares what experts commonly see. 'Women often find body image issues with their nose, face, waist, breasts or arms,' she says. 'Men find body image issues with their muscles, including biceps or shoulders.'

WHAT TO LOOK OUT FOR?

'Look out for words or phrases like "size zero", a fixation on weight loss, for anyone who has an aversion to food or seems to be starving themselves, or repeatedly saying:

- 'I need to be thin'
- 'My nose looks too big'
- 'I feel bloated and heavy'
- 'I need to lose weight'
- 'My arms look too big'
- 'My waist/hips look too broad'

Also, there are problem areas even with some strict diets — paleo diets, keto diets and intermittent fasting. Sometimes patients also show absolute aversion to foods where they absolutely don't eat or develop a psycho-somatic aversive reactions to foods.'

EATING DISORDERS: MYTHS AND FACTS
Smriti Joshi

• **Myth**: Having an eating disorder is a choice.

People often label anorexic behaviour as dissatisfaction with one's appearance and being anxious about it prompted by thoughts to attain perfect bodies and appearances. The association between body dissatisfaction and eating disorders can sometimes lead people to mistakenly believe that eating disorders are prompted by vanity and represent a lifestyle choice to attain body ideals.

Fact: Eating disorders are serious and potentially life-threatening mental illnesses and not just attempts to diet or look a certain way. An individual suffering from an eating disorder can experience severe disturbances in their behaviour around eating, exercising and related self-harm because of distortions in their thoughts and emotions and also gives rise to co-morbidities in both physical and mental health areas like physical fatigue and gastrointestinal (GI) tract issues or depression and anxiety.

The development of an eating disorder is an individual pathway, where genetic and personality vulnerabilities interact with social and environmental triggers.

• **Myth**: Eating disorders cannot be treated.

Fact: Eating disorders can be treated and managed though for some people, the process of recovering from an eating disorder can be long and challenging, as it often requires a multi-speciality approach. People with eating disorders require treatment for the underlying psychological issues and the impact on physical health. Treatment early in the development of the disorder can reduce the duration and severity of the illness. Yet, despite their seriousness, with the right treatment and support there is hope for recovery and improved quality of life at all stages of illness.

• **Myth**: Eating disorders are developed to gain attention, or is a phase that will get over soon.

This is one myth that actually reflects the beliefs about eating disorders amongst the general public and leads to delay in receiving the much-needed help.

Fact: An eating disorder is a serious mental illness. It is not a phase and it will not be resolved without treatment and support. Individuals with eating disorders are not being greedy for attention. In fact, due to the nature of an eating disorder a person may go to great extents to keep their conditions under wraps and disguise or deny their behaviour, or may not even recognise that there is anything wrong.

• **Myth**: Eating disorders only affect the affluent or middle class females and often only teenagers

Fact: Eating disorders can impact anyone across cultures, socio-economic status or genders. Research shows that the peak age of onset for anorexia nervosa is between 13-18 years.[95] It is wrong to presume that it impacts only women and those from the affluent or middle class. Population studies indicate that males form 25 per cent of those diagnosed with eating disorders.[96]

High-risk groups are:

- People into specific professions like modelling, dancing, or acting.
- Individuals suffering from disorders like thyroid or PCOD

- Individuals experiencing high levels of stress
- People who have other mental illnesses, such as anxiety or depression

• **Myth**: You can tell by looking at someone that they have an eating disorder.

Fact: The general public may often hold this belief that people with eating disorders may appear unwell and wasted. Many people with eating disorders look healthy yet may be extremely ill.

• **Myth**: Eating Disorders are about food or diets.

A commonly held belief about eating disorder amongst individuals with eating disorder or their families/caregivers is that eating disorders are about food, and are surprised when I inform them that eating disorders have little to do with food or dieting etc

Fact: It's not about just food or dieting. There is a larger problem, potentially a co-morbid condition or associated disorder.

The thoughts, behaviour or feelings around the food, or weight, or quantity of food are all signs of a larger problem. I also make sure clients are receiving the right medical help they may need for any other co-morbid disorder or any associated physical health issues. With most clients, the first step in getting help is to help them find the underlying issues, while also working on breaking the vicious cycle of the thoughts-feelings-negative coping strategies and symptoms. Adherence to therapy is a barrier as sometimes it can take months to years and more than technique of therapy it takes an empathetic, reassuring and non-judgemental therapist, a lot of motivational support and proactiveness on the therapist's part to help clients move towards recovery.

MYTHS AND FACTS ABOUT BODY IMAGE DISORDER
Pragya Lodha

- It's a myth that eating fats and carbs is bad for health: In fact, fats have a cardiac-protective value and carbs provide energy. All nutrients are needed in an apt and balanced amount.

- It's a myth that being overweight is always unhealthy: Lot of overweight people are fit and sometimes fitter than people who weigh less. Being healthy, active and having good stamina is important and can be established irrespective of being heavy. Many people with ED are not overweight, but actually unhappy or even depressed.

- It's a myth that one has to lose weight to feel body positive: It is not true, feeling body positive is to accept the body you have and rather focus on being healthy than on just losing weight.

- It's a myth that you need to be a certain size and shape to look pretty: Looking pretty is irrespective of shape size, colour and weight. It is a matter of perception. Being pretty is not a function of external appearance but internal understanding and being. Everyone can be their own pretty and beautiful in their own ways.

- It's a myth that body shaming can be healthy and motivational for weight loss: Body shaming is not acceptable and is derogatory in all ways to the other person. Motivating someone to lose weight is a matter of health choice that should be done in a respectful way, if at all, while respecting their privacy. There can be positive and healthier ways to make better health choices rather than just focusing on weight loss.

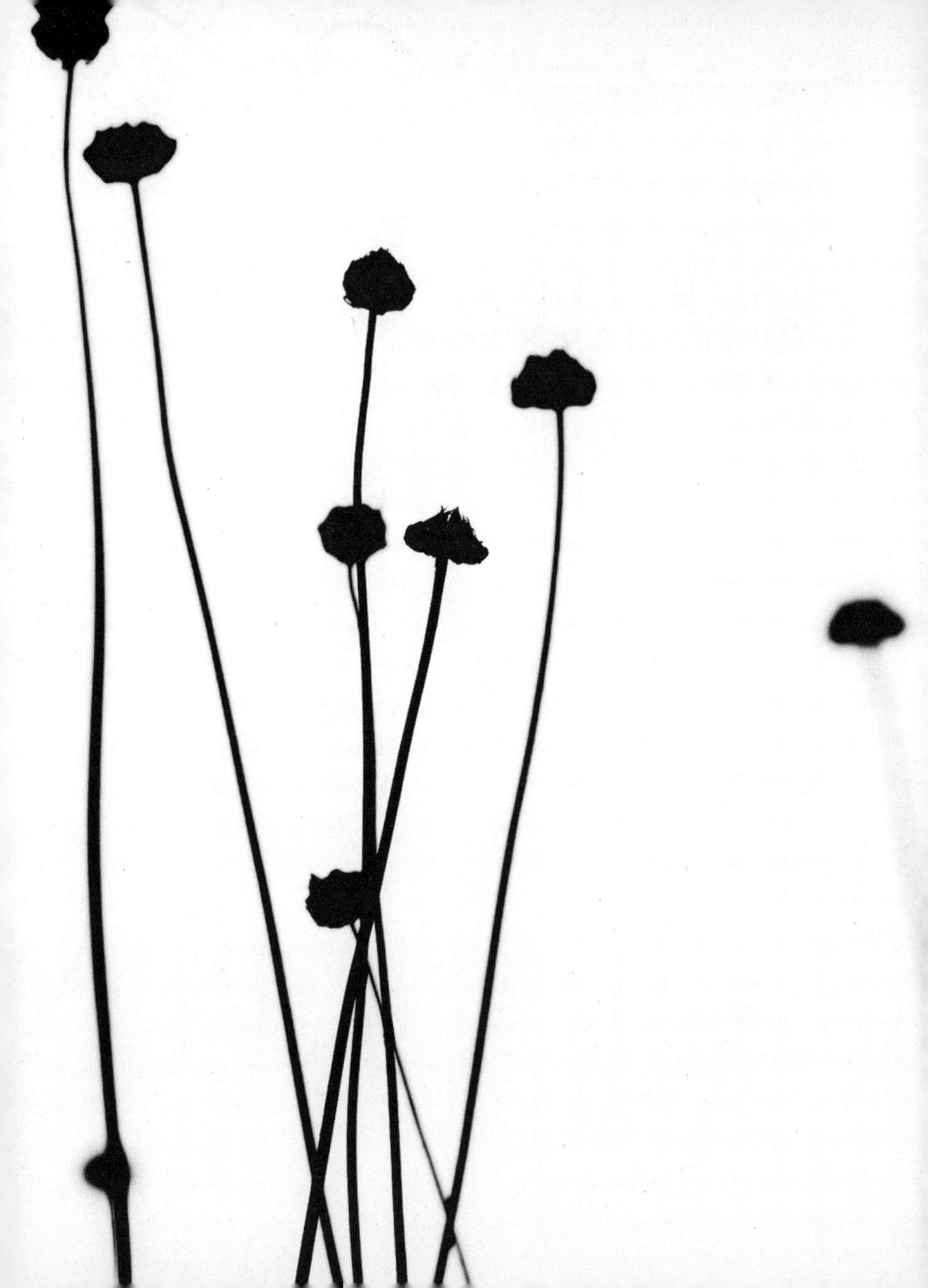

Chapter 18
PROMOTING MENTAL HEALTH IN THE STUDENT POPULATION BY DR SAMIR PARIKH AND KAMNA CHHIBBER

Mental health problems affect the youth as much as they affect adults. Recognising the need to work with this young population is imperative and it is critical that a preventive approach is adopted, which works by imparting life skills. Research has consistently pointed toward the need for equipping students with skills that allow them to cope effectively with stress, that provides mechanisms for identification of problems, and encourages help-seeking. This requires a deeper understanding of the issues and challenges which can compromise students' well-being and impact their state of mental health.

As adults we frequently view the problems faced by children and adolescents as emanating from factors that may not always be strongly correlated with the reasons they would have in mind themselves. A prominent reason for the disconnectedness between children and their parents (and other adults around them) arises from their feelings of not being understood or being misperceived and misinterpreted.

A significantly large proportion of the challenge students face occurs on account of the academic pressures they experience, which they feel pushes them to compromise on other facets of their life such as hobbies, extra-curricular activities, time with friends, relationships, or just relaxation. There is no denying that our existing educational system largely places a strong emphasis on academic proficiency.

The need to get high marks is stressed upon in schools as well as at homes. For many it is also reinforced, at times consciously and at other times through the inferences they draw from communication that happens around them, that without these high percentages of marks they would be of no good to themselves, their lives or society. As a consequence, students internalise an understanding of themselves and evaluate their goodness on the parameter of how well they are doing in their academic pursuits. Some gain recognition for their accomplishments in extra-curricular and sport-related activities. But at the back of their minds the need to excel in academics still persists. In this process, often the needs of a large majority of the student population do not tend to get addressed.

What also gets missed in this sprint towards gaining marks and maintaining a set standard of educational accomplishments is the focus on imparting life skills that allow them to cope with problems, manage their thoughts and emotions, make healthy choices and live a life with a focus on well-being that promotes their mental health.

Working with students via various programmes under the Fortis School Mental Health Program has highlighted the effectiveness of certain approaches. The team comprising mental health experts has been mindful of the significant shortage of mental health experts to help work with the large number of people who would benefit from the utilisation of mental health services. The work we want to outline has proven to be efficacious, cost-effective and culminated in better understanding

as well as the promotion of well-being and mental health. The emphasis is on the development of skills and tackling of problems at an early stage to prevent the development of a mental health illness on account of situational, psychological or emotionally driven vectors.

Following are a few highlighted approaches that prove effective.

UTILISING PEER INFLUENCE TO PROMOTE LIFE SKILLS

Peer relationships tend to be one of the most important aspects of an adolescent's life, as they seek friendship and companionship with others. They learn a large part of their culture from their peers, who are a source of comparison as well as validation for most young people. The comparisons that occur contribute to the adolescent's developing sense of self. Adolescents respond well to the encouragement and push received from their peers to try out a behaviour or an activity. Concurrently, they are likely to take their cue and are more easily influenced than those who are older than them. They can be influenced to enact negative behaviours, but that influence can also be utilised to promote positive, prosocial and altruistic behaviours.

Social influence can be used to create a cohesive way of responding when the group identifies with each other — an attribute which is prominent in schools as students do identify with each other and their cohort. Encouraging prosocial behaviours and their demonstration is known to promote altruism. Children who view positive, prosocial behaviours are likely to act helpfully as well on their own part. For example, the Fortis Pro-social Peer Moderator Programme involves an application-based learning of life skills wherein students themselves become peer trainers and positive role models, in turn helping other children in their schools learn healthier forms of coping. Simply teaching a skill-set, giving a talk or a lecture, or making them read or study a particular chapter is not the most helpful strategy, when it comes to life skills.

Young
MENTAL HEALTH

This programme involves imparting skills through six modules, namely Media Literacy, Risk Behaviour Management, Study and Exam Skills, Aggression Management, Gender Sensitisation and Caring for the Environment. The process involves training a small subset of the student population from the senior grades to become peer trainers for other students at their school premises. The training is facilitated in the presence of teacher moderators who provide the required support while programmes are conducted on school premise. The training for a module, for instance on Gender Sensitisation would involve helping students develop an experiential understanding of what gender is, what gender roles are, how they develop, how stereotypes and prejudices are internalised, critically think about how these are communicated and also developing ways to effectively respond to them, as well as build and nurture skills like empathy and assertiveness. This is done through the medium of videos, activities, role plays, and other methods that allow students to connect with the lived reality of these component elements.

Since the commencement of the program in 2012, the team at Fortis has trained more than 8,000 peer moderators. Students have shown great enthusiasm and innovation in communicating the messages they have learnt from the trainings they have undergone to other students at their respective schools. We have observed that when students are encouraged to actually interact with peers and train them, they take on immense responsibility and demonstrate enormous commitment to the objectives of the program.

MENTAL HEALTH ADVOCACY FOR THE YOUTH THROUGH

THE YOUTH

Mental health needs more voices. It needs greater reach. There is a requirement for greater engagement in ways that hold meaning and value for the youth. Another programme, the Fortis Young Mental Health Advocates programme engages with 20 young people in the age range of 15-21 years, who have a passion as well as a vision for mental health, demonstrate motivation, willingness and zeal to speak about various topics that relate to mental health.

Launched in 2019, our group of advocates, MindSpeakers2019, have worked dedicatedly on topics like studies, exam anxiety, suicide prevention, body image issues, bullying, to name a few, through the year. They have utilised varying platforms, including social media, newspapers, blogs, and workshops, to reach an increasing number of people about aspects relating to the topic they were working on for the month.

Their language is the language of the youth, making them relatable. They have been able to connect with the young population with greater ease, encouraging people to be more cognisant of what affects them, how they can take care of themselves, and when they should be reaching out for help, while also directing people to the right resources for support.

CREATING A MOVEMENT FOR BULLY-TO-BUDDY

The problem of bullying has been prevalent for decades. School and college students have experienced bullying in many formats over the years. When you step into a school and talk to students, or when children and adolescents reach us in out-patient departments, they often speak about the negative impact that episodes of bullying have had on them. A bigger concern for a large number of them involves lack of understanding and knowledge of the ways to tackle and address the issue.

A survey conducted by our team with over 1,000 students[97] revealed that 41 per cent of the students had experienced bullying themselves or seen someone else being bullied in their school. Sixty per cent students expressed that their friends and peers rarely or never stand up to a bully and these remain unreported to school authorities. Sixty-four per cent students were uninformed about the existence of a bullying prevention policy at their school.

The results obtained by our survey indicated the dire need for the creation and implementation of a programme that addresses the problem of bullying at a school-wide level. Addressing students alone, equipping them with the skills to be able to tackle instances of bullying, or dealing with the aftermath of the event alone was not going to be sufficient. This prompted us to design the Fortis Bully-to-Buddy programme which is a 100-day long programme that provides students with skills, addresses bystanders, and promotes working with the person who bullies. It also propagates and supports the creation of school-wide policies, supporting the school in the implementation of the same.

As its primary objective, the programme aims to sensitise schools and parents about bullying, helping take steps towards creating a 'bully-free' school, based on direct training of the students themselves. In the process, we create anti-bullying squads within the schools which involves students who are trained to identify the situation where bullying is occurring and enacting a simple act — standing with the person who is bullied in her or his support.

IMPORTANCE OF TRAINING FOR TEACHERS AND STAFF

AT SCHOOLS

Students spend a large proportion of their day at school, interacting with their peers and engaging with the staff and teachers in the school. Given the context of this reality, it is beneficial that training be provided to both teaching and non-teaching staff within schools on various aspects relating to mental health. This allows for the creation of spaces for conversations and engagement with mental health-related issues, normalising it within the culture of the school, encouraging students and staff to speak and share experiences without feeling shame, guilt or being ridiculed or castigated for their situation.

With this end in mind we have designed the Mental Health Curriculum, providing teachers specific guidelines through the medium of structured modules which can be introduced within the classrooms in a format that is most conducive to the pre-existing school environment. Accompanied by a manual, this training programme is being implemented in schools across the country, providing critical information to the staff, enabling them to provide the right kind of information, knowledge and support to students. In essence, the curriculum looks to focus on five key aspects, namely, understanding what mental health and mental health-related illnesses are, gaining information about stigma and breaking it, looking at aspects relating to building resilience and imparting life skills, and integrating well-being into the classroom. It is imperative that the staff be aware of the ways in which these can be spoken about, the right information that needs to be communicated as well as the ways in which students can be supported through the challenges they face, while providing them with the right resources for seeking help.

CREATING RESOURCES FOR HELP-SEEKING

Young
MENTAL HEALTH

Encouraging youth to seek help is critical. Often they and their families, including other adults surrounding them, tend to be inadequately informed about mental health related issues, how they occur, the ways in which they can be treated and more particularly what would be the right resources to seek help from. According to statistics[98], worldwide 70 per cent of the young people and adults do not seek treatment for mental health related concerns even when it is needed. In such a scenario it is necessary that they be directed towards the right resources and there be adequate information available about the same.

Early identification and intervention for mental health related problems are recognised as important intervening mechanisms. The lack of understanding and delaying seeking of intervention can lead to the worsening of concerns, making problems more resistant to treatment. At the same time, it is important to give due importance to the burden that mental health treatments can create given the longevity of the treatment duration. As a result, it is important to find ways to support the youth in a manner that they do not consider financially draining, as a viable medium for seeking help and can be easily reached in case they face a crisis.

Keeping this in mind we launched the Fortis 24x7 helpline (+918376804102) in 2013. The helpline has been running successfully, providing intervention services to individuals who are experiencing a mental health related concern. This helpline is run by our team of trained psychologists and receives over 100 calls on an average every day, from all across the country. The USP is the availability of speakers in multiple languages and 24/7 coverage.

If you or someone you know wants to reach out for help, please do not hesitate.

Young
MENTAL HEALTH

FIVE TIPS TO DEAL WITH EXAM-RELATED STRESS

Focus on inculcating the right study skills
There are specific, validated ways of studying that can be helpful. This includes ensuring you work in a clutter-free work space, that you keep only a single book in front of you, sit and work on a table and not your bed and remove all your gadgets.

- Study for 45 minutes and take a five minute break before you return to studying.
- Utilise mnemonics and highlighting as tools to aid learning and make sure you make your own notes.
- Revise using the 1,2,7,15,30 day rule which leads to maximum retention of information.

Test yourself to build your confidence
Create a habit of testing yourself regularly. Often students develop intense anxiety about being tested and can experience feeling blank on the day of the examination. Utilising self-tests as a tool to build confidence is helpful. It also allows you to determine the robustness of your learning and helps you understand which areas you need to work more on in terms of understanding concepts or memorising information.

FIVE TIPS TO DEAL WITH EXAM-RELATED STRESS

A balanced lifestyle is critical to academic success
Studying and doing well in an examination is possible if you maintain a balanced lifestyle. Being cooped up in your room with your books will not reduce stress. Instead, it is important to go out, meet friends, eat well, sleep according to your exam schedule, avoid caffeine and also exercise to ensure you manage the stress well.

Remember taking exams is a life skill
Treat examinations as teaching moments in life which aid you in building the right life skills. They enable understanding of time management, decision-making and problem-solving, besides testing your knowledge of a subject. Keep this in mind and remember that one bad exam will not ruing your life. Instead it is important to understand where you erred to ensure you do better in the next one. Comparing yourself to others — how well they did or how much they study or the number of extra sheets they used in the exam are of no value as they do nothing to contribute towards you achieving a better result.

Parents must play a supportive role
Parents can often feel equally anxious about their children's examinations. Maintaining their own calm is important to ensure they can offer the right support in helping their child lead a balanced life that reduces the levels of stress they experience during examinations. It is crucial to remember that each child can have his or her own areas of expertise which would be their strengths and they would do well in their lives by utilising these skills. Comparing, nagging and being critical or hostile do not help in any way and only serve to build the pressure of exams.

Young
MENTAL HEALTH

IN THEIR OWN WORDS: YOUNG MENTAL HEALTH ADVOCATE YASH SHAH

Yash Shah is an 18 year old from Bengaluru, who is studying for a BSc Hons in Psychology at CHRIST (Deemed to be University) School of Business Studies and Social Sciences. He was a student mental health advocate associated with the Fortis Young Mental Health Advocate programme and wants to spread awareness about mental health-related issues.

AMRITA: What led to your interest in mental health?

YASH SHAH: I was made more aware about mental health and mental illnesses throughout my 11th and 12th grade as I was familiarised with the basics of psychology as a subject. My psychology teacher in school — a major source of inspiration for me was a psychologist herself. She'd share lots of stories about her experiences and that motivated me to understand the grey areas of human behaviour, mental health and illnesses.

However, I realised the actual degree of the issue of mental health and the lack of its awareness in our country, when I visited the Stepping-Stones Centre, an institution that uses intervention techniques to treat behavioural and developmental disorders in children, for a project from school.

My time spent with a seven-year-old child belonging to the Autism Spectrum reinforced the drive within me to understand and contribute to the field of mental health. I was also lucky to have the opportunity to intern with Fortis Healthcare during a summer break. Here, I was given practical exposure and was introduced to expressive art therapy, group therapy and various case studies in detail. The programs shed light on the prevailing ignorance and stigma towards mental health which I strongly believe must be eradicated.

AMRITA: Can you describe what the Youth Mental Health Advocate programme has been like — what has your experience been like? Did you enjoy it?

YASH SHAH: The Youth Mental Health programme has been very insightful. It has helped me become more aware about different aspects of mental health that I didn't know of. It's taught me how to be sensitive while creating awareness through different platforms. We've had some great mentors over the past few months who helped us expand our reach and presence to create a bigger impact. I enjoyed being a part of this initiative.

AMRITA: What was the biggest take-away?

YASH SHAH: My biggest take-away was the amount I was able to learn with the help of this programme. Working with 20 young and motivated minds helped me gain a new perspective about different issues and how they could be approached.

AMRITA: How easy/difficult is it to talk to peers or friends and family about issues to do with mental health and mental illness?

YASH SHAH: I think one positive impact that social media has on its users is

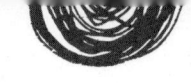

Young
MENTAL HEALTH

that it makes us aware, although sometimes it can be misleading. However, the way mental health and mental illnesses are being depicted and spoken about seems to be in a positive and empowering context. This depiction is slowly but surely being acknowledged, understood and accepted by people of all age groups. Therefore, communicating about such issues in general has become relatively easier.

In my case, I've always found it easy to discuss and debate on such issues with my friends and family. My friends and I can openly, freely and honestly talk about what we believe, feel, etc. I'm also able to discuss such issues with my parents without much hesitation. Although it may take more time and effort to explain issues like these since they themselves haven't had enough exposure to them, they've always lent an ear and have never been reluctant to understand and learn more about mental health and illness.

AMRITA: Can you share a bit about your social media posts?

YASH SHAH: The first three were in relation to exam stress and the fourth is a post on body image. We conducted a poll on different behaviours that are seen during exams. It was very interactive, and all the young advocates gathered lots of responses.

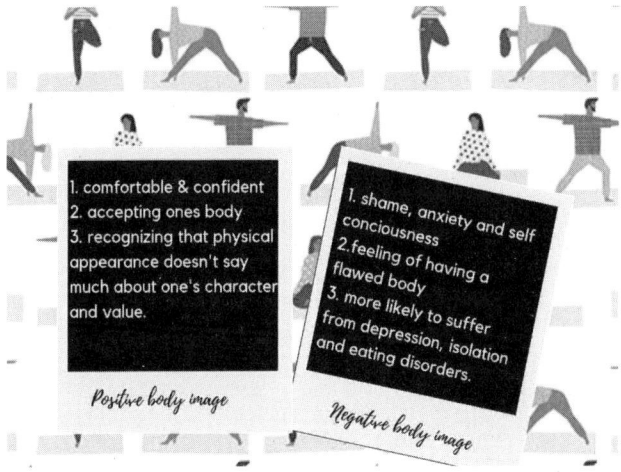

Image Courtesy: @chooseyourhappiness

The fourth picture was created in collaboration with three other young advocates. We run an Instagram page together called @chooseyourhappiness. We were targeting the issue of body image, something that I can personally relate to. I myself have been through positive body transformation so it was refreshing to create awareness about health positivity.

AMRITA: Did you think that folks at your high school were open in talking about mental health? What made it easier or harder to have these conversations?

YASH SHAH: Yes, to some extent they were. I've had good conversations with my peers and even my juniors at high school about mental health. I believe what makes it easy or hard to talk about such things, which are so personal, is trust. The fear of being judged makes it harder to talk about mental health. A mutual

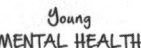
MENTAL HEALTH

understanding and a non-judgemental attitude between both the parties can facilitate a healthy conversation about mental health. What also makes a difference is knowing that having a conversation about mental health is normal. It's like talking about a headache or a sprain. It's imperative we realise mental health as a subject neither needs to be hyped up nor pushed under the carpet, rather it needs to be cleansed of its layers of misconceptions and stigma.

AMRITA: What does your family think of your interest in mental health and mental illness and do you find it easy to have these conversations at home?

YASH SHAH: I've been conversing about mental health and illnesses with my parents ever since I started learning psychology in 11th grade. At first, they saw it as an unexplored territory which made it difficult for them to understand and appreciate. But this attitude changed and over time they were able to recognise the worth of this topic. This shift in their attitude was possible only because they were ready to strike a conversation with me. They never failed to keep an open mind and question me whenever they felt there was a clash with their own perspectives. I aspire to contribute to this field in the future and my parents are happy and excited about it.

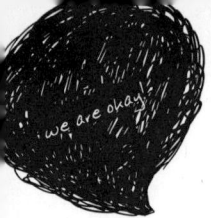

HELPLINES IN INDIA

ALL-INDIA	VANDREVALA FOUNDATION	1800-233-3330/ 0261-2662700/ 1860-266-2345	24 by 7 EMAIL: help@vandrevalafoundation.com
	ICALL HELPLINE	022-25521111	MON-SAT: 8 am to 10 pm/ EMAIL: icall@tiss.edu/ http://icallhelpline.org/
	FORTIS HOSPITAL NATIONAL HELPLINE	91-8376804102	24 by 7 / Multilingual
BANGALORE	SAHAI	080-25497777	
CHENNAI	JEEVAN SUICIDE PREVENTION HOTLINE	044-2656 4444	
	SNEHA	044-2464 0050	EMAIL: help@snehaindia.org
DELHI	SANJIVINI SOCIETY FOR MENTAL HEALTH	24311918, 243118883	EMAIL: sanjivini1971@gmail.com
	SNEHI	9582208181	10 am to 10 pm Daily
GANGTOK	SIKKIM HELPLINE NUMBER	1800-3453225 / 03592-202111	
HYDERABAD	ONE LIFE	78930 78930	
KOCHI	MAITHRI	91-484-2540530	
KOLKATA	SERVE	9830785060	
	DEFEAT DEPRESSION	9830027975	
	CLIPPINGS	98300 27976	
MUMBAI	SINGING SOULZ	9892003868	

	SAMARITANS	84229 84528/ 84229 84529 / 84229 84530	3-9 PM (all days) EMAIL: talk2samaritans@gmail.com You can call and speak anonymously and confidentially, or visit the centre for a personal meeting in Mumbai, with a prior appointment. Address:402, Jasmine, Opp Kala Kendra, Dadasaheb Phalke Road, Dadar(E), Mumbai 400014
NAGPUR	Nagpur Suicide Prevention Helpline	8888817666	

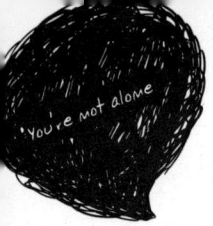

ACKNOWLEDGEMENTS

AMRITA

My deepest gratitude and acknowledgements for each and every contributor, as well as the stellar The Health Collective team and tribe. We wouldn't be here without you, without your stories, wisdom and courage. It's been such a transformative experience to work with you in this space over the past three years.

I am so grateful to Meera, my dear friend and co-author, who took up this challenging project with flair, enthusiasm and her characteristic dedication (and humility!). It's been a privilege to work with and learn from you. We've sure come a long way since Hudson Lines; I'm always going to be thankful that you handled some of our experiences (not to mention delinquent behaviour) with so much grace and tact. Thanks a ton Manini and Nithanth as well for your illustrations!

Thank you so much to Dr Amit Sen, for the past decade and a half of interviews, (from a news channel to digital!) leading up all the way up to 2020. I'm more than grateful for your time, expertise, grace and words, including the foreword to this book.

Thank you again to Kamna Chhibber and Dr Samir Parikh for your passion, the interviews, and for giving me a chance to interact with your Youth Mental Health advocates. Thank you to Yash and Ananya for sharing your time and some of your thoughts.

To the incredible artists: Ishita Mehra, Solo, Oz, Kishore Mohan and Adwaita Das, a heart-felt thank you. I am in awe of your talent and your work has elevated this book.

Anwesh, your words are so moving, elegant, and brave that I can only laud your courage and eloquence and thank you. Huge thanks to Anant for connecting and inspiring us as well. Thank you to the powerhouses Paras and Pattie for making the time for this interview though it couldn't be face-to-face, beyond our initial chats. Your work and your teams' work couldn't be more inspiring and illuminating. And that goes double for iCall and Tanuja, thanks for your interview with Sukanya Sharma; huge thanks also to Manisha Chachra for sharing your story with us.

Sukanya, you have been such a delight to work with, thanks for all the effort and wherewithal at nearly the last second (!) huge appreciation. Devanik Saha, thank you for your hard work in collating the research we used and will be sharing on our site; Vandita, for all your support including on some of the tailwinds, and Mohit Dhingra for energising so many of us with your ideas, and for your piece in this book. Ilina Acharya for all your boundless help with the references and proof-reading, as well as for your patience!

Thank you to the kindest and most understanding of editors, Himanjali, and Rahul and the whole team at Simon & Schuster India for taking a punt on this entire Mindscape series, including Sayantan for his keen (and empathetic) eye, Abhay and Shobhita for all the tireless work, as well as to Mridu for her stellar cover and design work!

Thanks to the wonderful Amartya for being a legal eagle and for all the positive support and validation (despite the general state of the world), Karan, we wouldn't have reached this stage without your enthusiasm and wisdom and friendship, thanks for everything.

To my whole family, especially Mum and Suren, love you loads and can't thank you enough for being in my life and supporting all kinds of flights of fancy. Dad, wish you were around for an unfiltered conversation; I'll always be grateful for the love and no holds-barred attitude to life, truth and the things that matter. And last but not least, the secret weapon that is Abhishek, who has been beyond supportive even when faced with a tirade of self-doubt, existential angst or endless reasons why something might not work.

MEERA

Who would imagine that I would be co-authoring a book with Amrita my wonderful friend and flat mate from 20 years ago! I still remember our long deep conversations in the narrow balcony of our shady Hudson lines flat and the mad late night cycle rickshaw rides through civil lines ... Wow, we have both come such a long way and it has been an amazing blessing to be re-united with you now to share this beautiful journey together... I have learnt so much from you through this writing process and it's been fantastic collaborating with you on this project in a subject so close to my heart.

I dedicate this book to my most beautiful and amazing children Manini and Nithanth.

Manini, I feel so lucky to see you grow into this beautiful, graceful and thoughtful young woman and Nithanth, I absolutely enjoy how free spirited you are, so individualistic in your thinking, with a wise old heart! What a privilege and blessing it has been to be your 'Amma'- thank you both for being you!

Special thanks to all the wonderful children and families that I have worked with over the years. I have been touched by your lives and it has been my honour to witness your journey.

My utmost gratitude to my 'core' family for all your love and support: my 'Amma': Indira, for being my role model in teaching me the value of hard work, honesty and discipline, my 'Appa': Haran, for instilling in me the drive to pursue my passion and for your ever-loving faith in me, my 'Anna': Murali, for your unflinching support and for your valuable advice that I can always count on and my 'Mamma':

Margaret, for inspiring me to live a life of courage and commitment by example. I miss you my 'Dada' : Niranjan, I will forever remember your loving smile and your infectious laugh. You will remain in my heart always.

A shout out to all my old and gold friends in Delhi- Meera Piyush, Subhashim and Megha, my wonderful new tribe of friends in Bangalore and to all my extended family members in Bangalore, Gurgaon, New Jersey and Pennsylvania for all your cheer and support.

And above all, my deepest gratitude and love to my wonderful husband, Nivedith, for being present throughout the process of writing this book with your unstinting, unconditional- love, faith and support that fuels my dreams and me ...

Notes

1 Rajeev Radhakrishnan and Chitaranjan Andrade,'Suicide: An Indian Perspective', *Indian Journal of Psychiatry* Vol. 54, no.4 (2012): 304-319. (DOI: 10.4103/0019-5545.104793)
2 Ibid.
3 Suicide Prevention Helplines. (http://www.healthcollective.in/suicide-prevention-helplines/)
4 'Mental Health Atlas 2011', World Health Organization, last accessed 15 March 2020.
(https://www.who.int/mental_health/evidence/atlas/profiles/ind_mh_profile.pdf)
5 MHRD (2005), 'Action Plan for Inclusive Education of Children and Youth with Disabilities', last accessed 15 March 2020.
(http://www.education.nic.in)
J.D. Singh, 'Inclusive Education in India – Concept, Need and Challenges', *Scholarly Research Journal* vol. 3, no. 13 (2016): 3222–3232. (http://www.srjis.com/issues_data?issueId=9)
6 Bharath Srikala and Kumar K.V. Kishore, 'Empowering adolescents with life skills education in schools — School mental health program: Does it Work?', *Indian J Psychiatry* 52(4) 2010 Oct-Dec: 344–349.
(https://www.ncbi.nlm.nih.gov/pmc/articles/PMC3025161/)
7 Stephan Ecks, Christine Kupfer, 'What is strange is that we don't have more children coming to us: A habitography of child psychiatrists and scholastic pressure in Kolkata, India', *Social Science and Medicine* 143, (October 2015): 336–342.
(https://www.sciencedirect.com/science/article/abs/pii/S0277953614007801)
8 G. Gururaj, et al, 'National Mental Health Survey of India, 2015-16: Prevalence, patterns and outcomes', National Institute of Mental Health and Neuro Sciences, NIMHANS Publication No. 129 (2016). (http://indianmhs.nimhans.ac.in/Docs/Report2.pdf)
9 Ibid.
10 Rakhi Dandona, et al., 'Gender differentials and state variations in suicide deaths in India: the Global Burden of Disease Study 1990–2016', *The Lancet 3*, no.10 (September 11, 2018). (https://doi.org/10.1016/S2468-2667(18)30138-5)
11 'National Mental Health Survey of India, 2015-16', (NIMHANS, Bengaluru: 2016).
12 Ibid
13 R. Parikh, et al., 'It is like a mind attack: stress and coping among urban school-going adolescents in India', *BMC Psychology* 7, 31 (2019). (https://bmcpsychology.biomedcentral.com/articles/10.1186/s40359-019-0306-z)
14 Ibid.
15 Mohit Dhingra, 'It's Time To Pay Attention: India's Biggest Public Health Crisis is Suicide', Health Collective, 6 October 2019. (http://www.healthcollective.in/2019/10/its-time-to-pay-attention-indias-biggest-public-health-crisis-is-suicide/)
16 Lakshmi Vijayakumar et al., 'Suicide in India: a complex public health tragedy in need of a plan', *The Lancet Public Health* 3,10 (2018): e459-e460. (DOI: https://doi.org/10.1016/S2468-2667(18)30142-7)
17 Dandona et al., 'Gender Differentials and State Variations'.
18 Shreevatsa Nevatia, 'Why Is It So Hard To Find Good Mental Healthcare In India?', HuffPost India, retrieved 3 November 2019. (https://www.huffingtonpost.in/entry/good-mental-healthcare-in)
19 'Annual Report 2018-2019'. (https://wcd.nic.in/sites/default/files/WCD%20ENGLISH%202018-19.pdf)
20 Vikram Patel, et al., 'Suicide Mortality in India: A Nationally Representative Survey', *The Lancet* 379, no. 9834 (2012). (DOI: https://doi.org/10.1016/S0140-6736(12)60606-0)
21 Randy Auerbach, et al., 'One in Three College Freshmen Worldwide Reports Mental Health Disorder', American Psychological Association, 13 September 2018. (https://www.apa.org/news/press/releases/2018/09/freshmen-mental-health)
22 'Ask The Experts: Understanding ADD and ADHD', The Health Collective, 5 July 2018. (http://www.healthcollective.in/2018/07/ask-the-experts-understanding-add-and-adhd/)
23 Ibid.
24 Dr Amit Sen, 'Ask the Experts: Bullying and School Kids', The Health Collective, 22 April 2018. (http://www.healthcollective.in/2018/04/ask-the-experts-bullying-and-school-kids/)
25 'The Freedom Series: My Journey'. (www.healthcollective.in/2018/08/the-freedom-series-my-journey/)
26 Manisha Chachra, 'Suicide Prevention Day: Let's Talk, Connect', The Health Collective, 10 September 2018. (http://www.healthcollective.in/2018/09/suicide-prevention-day-talk/)

27 Devanik Saha, 'A Student Commits Suicide Every Hour In India', IndiaSpend, 6 April 2017. (http://www.indiaspend.com/special-reports/a-student-commits-suicide-every-hour-in-india-3-85917)

28 Prachi Salve, 'Nearly 60 Million Indians Suffer from Mental Disorders', IndiaSpend, 2 September 2016. (http://www.indiaspend.com/cover-story/nearly-60-million-indians-suffer-from-mental-disorders-68507)

29 Kamna Chhibber, 'Suicide Prevention Day: Creating The Space to Seek Help', The Health Collective, 10 September 2018. (http://www.healthcollective.in/2018/09/suicide-prevention-day-creating-space-to-seek-help/)

30 Kamna Chhibber, 'Is Your Therapist Right For You?', The Health Collective, 30 April 2018. (http://www.healthcollective.in/2018/04/is-your-therapist-right-for-you/)

31 'India's Biggest Public Health Crisis Is Suicide', The Health Collective, 6 October 2019. (http://www.healthcollective.in/2019/10/its-time-to-pay-attention-indias-biggest-public-health-crisis-is-suicide/)

32 For more, visit http://www.c3india.org/youthbolfindings

33 https://nonchalentyeteuphoric.wordpress.com/2019/06/16/the-three-players/

34 P.P. Gonsalves, et al., 'What are young Indians saying about mental health? A content analysis of blogs on the It's Ok To Talk website', *BMJ* Open Vol. 9 no. 6 (2019): e028244. (DOI: doi:10.1136/bmjopen-2018-028244.)

35 https://itsoktotalk.in

36 P.P. Gonsalves, et al., 'Design and Development of the 'POD Adventures' Smartphone Game: A Blended Problem-Solving Intervention for Adolescent Mental Health in India', Frontiers. 7:238 (2019). (DOI: 10.3389/fpubh.2019.00238.)

37 'The Power of 1.8 billion: Adolescents, Youth and the Transformation of the Future', United Nations Population Fund (2014), retrieved 28 August 2019. (https://www.unfpa.org/sites/default/ les/pub-pdf/EN-SWOP14-Report_FINAL-web.pdf)

38 V. Patel, et al., 'Mental Health of Young People: A Global Public-Health Challenge' *The Lancet* 369, no. 9569 (2017): 1302-1313. (DOI: 10.1016/s0140-6736(07)60368-7.)

39 'Dial iCall For Help: How The TISS-Housed Helpline Delivers', The Health Collective, 8 October 2019. (http://www.healthcollective.in/2019/10/dial-icall-for-help-how-the-tiss-housed-helpline-delivers/)

40 Kendra Cherry, 'Child Development Theories and Examples', Very Well Mind, updated 4 January 2020. (https://www.verywellmind.com/child-development-theories-2795068)

41 Charles E. Schaefer, Theresa F. DiGeronimo, *Ages and Stages: A Parent's Guide to Normal Childhood Development* (New York: Wiley, 2000)

42 James Marcia, Ruthellen Josselson, 'Eriksonian Personality Research and Its Implications for Psychotherapy', *Journal of Personality* vol. 8, no. 6 (2012). (DOI: 10.1111/jopy.12014.)

43 Pam Levine-Landheer, 'The Cycle of Development', *Transactional Analysis Journal* vol.12, no. 2 (1982):129- 139. (DOI: 10.1177/036215378201200207)

44 N. Tripathi, T.V. Sekher, 'Youth in India Ready for Sex Education? Emerging evidence from national surveys', *Plos one* vol. 8, no.8 (2013): e71584. (https://doi.org/10.1371/journal.pone.0071584)

45 Robert A Baron, *Introduction to Psychology* (Pearson, 2009)

46 Neeti Vijayakumar, '11 Amazing Indian Books to Take Children Through Sex Education and Puberty', The Better India, 22 April 2016. (https://www.thebetterindia.com/53187/11-books-sex-ed-puberty-teens-kids-indian/)

47 Rudi Dallos, Ros Draper, *An Introduction to Family Therapy: Systematic Theory and Practice* (Philadelphia, Penn: Open University Press, 2000).

48 Reena Nath, *Healing Room* (HarperCollins Publishers India, 2017)

49 Alan Carr, *Family Therapy: Concepts, Process and Practice* (New York: John Wiley & Sons, 2000).

50 Rudi Dallos, *An Introduction to Family Therapy: Systematic Theory and Practice*

51 Betty Carter, Monica McGoldrick, *The Changing family life cycle: a framework for family therapy* (Boston: Allyn and Bacon, 1989).

52 S. Kapadia, 'Adolescent-Parent Relationships in Indian and Indian Immigrant Families in the US: Intersections and Disparities', *Psychology and Developing Societies* vol. 20, no. 2 (2008): 257–275. (https://doi.org/10.1177/097133360802000207)

53 NG Preto, 'Transformation of the Family System during Adolescence', in *The Expanded Family Life Cycle: Individual, Family and Social Perspectives*, ed. B Carter & M McGoldrick (Boston: Allyn & Bacon, 1999), 274-286.

54 J . Byng-Hall, 'The Application of Attachment Theory to Understanding and Treatment in Family Therapy', in *Attachment across the life cycle*, ed. J.S. Hinde, P. Marris (New York, NY, US: Tavistock/Routledge, 1991),199–215.

55 Emilia Dowling and Elsie Osborne, ed., The Family and the School: *A Joint Systems Approach to Problems with Children* (New York: Routledge, 2019).

56 Alan Carr, 'The Evidence Base for Family Therapy and Systemic Interventions for Child-Focused Problems', *Journal of Family Therapy* Vol. 36, no. 2 (2014): 107–157. (https://www.lenus.ie/handle/10147/596078)

57 L. Lowenstein, *Creative Family Therapy Techniques: Play, Art, and Expressive Therapies to Engage Children in Family Sessions* (Toronto: Champion Press, 2010).

58 R. Nath, J. Craig, 'Practising family therapy in India: how many people are there in a marital subsystem?' *Journal of Family Therapy* vol.21 no. 4 (1999): 390–406. (doi: 10.1111/1467-6427.00127.)

59 D. L. Couchenour and K. Chrisman, *Families, Schools, and Communities: Together for Young Children.* (Belmont, CA: Wadsworth/Cengage Learning, 2014).

60 Janice H. Goodman, 'Perinatal depression and infant mental health', *Archives of Psychiatric Nursing* vol. 33, no. 3 (2019): 217–224. (https://doi.org/10.1016/j.apnu.2019.01.010)

61 Ivan Eisler, Mima Simic, et al., 'A pragmatic randomised multi-centre trial of multifamily and single family therapy for adolescent anorexia nervosa' *BMC* Psychiatry 16, 422 (2016). (https://doi.org/10.1186/s12888-016-1129-6)

62 Thapar, et al., 'Depression in Adolescents', *The Lancet* 379, 9820 (2012):1056-67. (DOI: 10.1016/S0140-6736(11)60871-4)

63 *Diagnostic and Statistical Manual of Mental Disorders: DSM-5.* (Arlington, VA: American) Psychiatric Association, 2017.

64 Ronald D. Siegel, *The Mindfulness Solution: Everyday Practices for Everyday Problems* (New York: Guilford Press, 2010).

65 Meghna Singhal, et al., 'Subclinical Depression in Urban Indian Adolescents: Prevalence, Felt Needs and Correlates', *Indian Journal of Psychiatry* Vol 58, no. 4 (2016): 394–402. (http://www.indianjpsychiatry.org/text.asp?2016/58/4/394/196727)

66 M.S. Clark, et al., 'Treatment of childhood and adolescent depression', *NCBI* 86,5 (2012): 442–448. (https://pubmed.ncbi.nlm.nih.gov/22963063/)

67 Ibid.

68 David Cottrell, 'Outcome Studies of Family Therapy in Child and Adolescent Depression', *Journal of Family Therapy* vol. 25, no. 4 (2003): 406–416. (https://doi.org/10.1111/1467-6427.00258)

69 S. Jiminez, et al., 'A mindfulness model of affect regulation and depressive symptoms: Positive emotions, mood regulation expectancies, and self-acceptance as regulatory mechanisms', *Elsevier* vol. 49, no. 6 (2010): 645–650. (DOI: 10.1016/j.paid.2010.05.041.)

70 R.D. Mckim, 'Rumination as a mediator of the effects of mindfulness: Mindfulness-based stress reduction (MBSR)', *Dissertation Abstracts International: Section B: The Sciences and Engineering*, 68(11-B), 7673 (2008). (https://psycnet.apa.org/record/2008-99100-247)

71 W. Kuyken, et al., 'Mindfulness-based cognitive therapy to prevent relapse in recurrent depression', *Journal of Consulting and Clinical Psychology* 76, 6 (2008): 966–978. (DOI: 10.1037/a0013786.)

72 M. Kerryann, 'Anxiety among High School Students in India: Comparisons across Gender, School Type, Social Strata, and Perceptions of Quality Time with Parents', *Australian Journal of Educational and Developmental Psychology* 10, (2010):18–31. (https://www.researchgate.net/publication/228639368)

73 Patty Wipfler and Tosha Schore, *Listen: Five Simple Tools to Meet Your Everyday Parenting Challenge* (Palo Alto, CA: Hand in Hand, 2016).

74 Sharan Salzberg, Lovingkindness: *The Revolutionary Art of Happiness* (Boston: Shambala, 2002).

75 Susanne Knappe, et al., 'Anxiety and Anxiety Disorders in Children and Adolescents: Developmental Issues and Implications', *Elsevier* vol. 32, no. 3 (2009): 483–524. (DOI: https://doi.org/10.1016/j.psc.2009.06.002)

76 L.M. Dufton, M.J. Dunn, et al., 'Anxiety and Somatic Complaints in Children with Recurrent Abdominal Pain and Anxiety Disorders', *Journal of Pediatric Psychology* 34, 2 (2008): 176–86. (DOI: https://doi.org/10.1093/jpepsy/jsn064.)

77 *Diagnostic and Statistical Manual of Mental Disorders*.

78 D.S. Pine, J. Grun, 'Childhood Anxiety: Integrating Developmental Psychopathology and Affective Neuroscience', *Journal of Child and Adolescent Psychopharmacoology* Vol 9. no. 1 (1999): 1-12. DOI: 10.1089/cap.1999.9.1.

79 Malgorzata Dabkowska, Agnieszka Dabkowska-Mika, 'Risk Factors of Anxiety Disorders in Children', *Psychiatria i Psychologia Kliniczna* 14, 2 (2014):127–129. (https://cdn.intechopen.com/pdfs/48919.pdf)

80 O.N. Velting, Nicole J. Setzer, et al., 'Update on and advances in assessment and cognitive-behavioral treatment of anxiety disorders in children and adolescents', *Professional Psychology: Research and Practice* 35,1 (2004). (DOI: IO.1031/0135-102R.15.1.42)

81 S. Hoffman, et al., 'The Effects of Mindfulness Based Therapy on Anxiety and Depression: A Meta-Analytic Review', *Journal of Consulting and Clinical Psychology* 78, 2 (2010): 69-83. (https://pubmed.ncbi.nlm.nih.gov/20350028/)

82 Jon Kabat-Zinn, *Wherever You Go, There You Are: Mindfulness Meditation in Everyday Life*, 2nd Ed. (New York, NY: Hachette Books, 2005).)

83 G.S. Ginsburg, 'The Child Anxiety Prevention Study: Intervention Model and Primary Outcomes', *Journal of Consulting and Clinical psychology* 77, 3 (2009): 580–587. (DOI: 10.1037/a0014486.)

84 A. Kumar, et al., 'The Need for Training Medical professionals in Child Sexual Abuse', *Journal of Psychosexual Health* Vol no. 1, 2 (2019): 192–194. (DOI: https://doi.org/10.1177/2631831819833618)

85 Vikram Patel, et al., 'Child Sexual Abuse in India: A Systematic Review', *Plos One* 13, no. 10 (2018): e0205086. (DOI: 10.1371/ journal.pone.0205086.

86 Edited excerpts from 'Overcoming an Eating Disorder', published on The Health Collective. (http://www.healthcollective.in/2016/09/your-story-overcoming-an-eating-disorder/)

87 Sivapriya Vaidyanath, et al., 'Eating Disorders: An Overview of Indian research', Indian Journal of Psychological Medicine Volume 41, no.4 (2019): 311-317. (DOI: 10.4103/IJPSYM.IJPSYM_461_18)

88 National Eating Disorder Association (NEDA), last accessed 12 April 2020. https://www.nationaleatingdisorders.org/about-us/our-work

89 Eating Disorder Statistics, Eating Disorder Help, last accessed 17 March 2020. https://www.mirror-mirror.org/eating-disorders-statistics.htm

90 'Eating Disorders', Psychology Today, last accessed 12 April 2020. https://www.psychologytoday.com/intl/conditions/ eating-disorders

91 'Body Image', NEDA, last accessed 12 April 2020. https://www.nationaleatingdisorders.org/body-image-0

92 Ibid.

93 'Statistics and Research on Eating Disorders', NEDA, last accessed 12 April 2020. https://www.nationaleatingdisorders.org/statistics-research-eating-disorders

94 Cameron Wilson, 'TikTok Is Filled With Pro-Eating Disorder Content', Buzzfeed, 17 February 2020. (https://www.buzzfeed.com/cameronwilson/tiktok-eating-disorder-videos-algorithm-for-you-page)

95 Nadia Micali, et al., 'Lifetime and 12-month prevalence of eating disorders amongst women in mid-life: a population- based study of diagnoses and risk factors', BMC Med 15, no. 12 (2017). (DOI: https://doi.org/10.1186/s12916-016-0766-4)

96 '*Statistics and Research on Eating Disorders*', NEDA

97 Rhythma Kaul, 'Bullies of the virtual world', Hindustan Times, 18 December 2016. (https://www.hindustantimes.com/health-and-fitness/bullies-of-the-virtual-world/story-RDPNLWeCgSNYO89RU2A7NI.html)

98 Claire Henderson, et al., 'Mental Illness Stigma, Help Seeking, and Public Health Programs', *AJPH* 103, no. 5 (2013): 777–780. (https://www.ncbi.nlm.nih.gov/pmc/articles/PMC3698814/)

MINDSCAPE SERIES

Real stories of dealing with depression
Young mental health
Age of Anxiety

NEXT IN THE MINDSCAPE SERIES: AGE OF ANXIETY
By Amrita Tripathi and Kamna Chhibber

Are we living through an Age of Anxiety? What should we make of all the new concerns, worries and fears amidst the uncertainty to do with Covid-19? It's time for a time-out – we'll listen to those who have lived and dealt with anxiety for years, and learned to heal. Equipping ourselves with the vocabulary we need, and fortified by expert insights and lessons from lived experiences, we'll be much better placed to take stock and reach out for help if we need to.